WAITING
FOR
ELI

A Father's Journey from Fear to Faith

WAITING
FOR
ELI

Chad Judice

Acadian House
PUBLISHING
Lafayette, Louisiana

Library of Congress Cataloging-in-Publication Data

Judice, Chad.
  Waiting for Eli : a father's journey from fear to faith / Chad Judice.
    p. cm.
  Includes bibliographical references and index.
  ISBN-13: 978-0-925417-65-7 (hardcover : alk. paper)
  ISBN-10: 0-925417-65-3 (hardcover : alk. paper) 1. Judice,
Eli, 2009–Health. 2. Spina bifida–Patients–Louisiana–Lafayette–
Biography. 3. Judice, Chad. 4. Spina bifida–Patients–Family
relationships. 5. Fathers of children with disabilities–Louisiana–
Lafayette–Biography. I. Title.
  RJ496.S74J83 2009
  618.92'73092--dc22
  [B]

                2009052688

♦ Published by Acadian House Publishing, Lafayette,
  Louisiana (Edited by Trent Angers)

♦ Cover design by Kevin Pontiff, Lafayette, Louisiana

♦ Printed by Sheridan Books, Chelsea, Michigan

Preface

'You've got to read this'

Sometime in the summer of 2009, I was in my office editing a book that was scheduled to go to press in the very near future. I was fully engaged with the project, as was most of my staff. We were plodding along, buried in work, and under considerable deadline pressure.

Then in strolls a teacher from a local high school, St. Thomas More, to drop off a manuscript written by one of her colleagues. She hands it to one of our office workers and talks to him about it for a few minutes. He promptly knocks on my door, enters my office, and announces:

"This lady from St. Thomas More just dropped this off and said to tell you, 'You've *got* to read this,' and that she knows you'll want to publish it once you do."

He went on to repeat some of what the visitor said about the book. I gathered it was written by a high school teacher named Chad Judice, whose wife was pregnant with a child with a dreaded birth defect, and that *everyone* who knew of them was praying for a miracle.

It sounded like a story with fairly good possibilities, but I wasn't interested in any new manuscripts at the time. We were under contract to produce two other books in short order and we had a dozen book proposals under consideration. There was too much on my plate already. I didn't need something else to think about.

However, for some reason, I didn't put the newly received manuscript in the stack "to be assigned to a reader," but instead it went into my stack of papers "to bring home and look at with fresh eyes in the morning."

So I bring the manuscript home and my wife recognizes

the name of the author. Turns out, he had been a student at a school where she taught when he was a youngster. She starts to peruse the pages and within twenty minutes she's in tears. An hour later, she's still reading and is in tears again. She declares:

"You've *got* to read this."

So that makes two people in the same day saying the same thing, urging me to make the time to look seriously at this story.

By now, I'm mildly interested and a little curious, but too worn out to read anything. My eyes are tired, my energy depleted. No way I'm reading anything else before I go to bed. It's after nine o'clock.

But the story beckons. I'm starting to wonder: *What's this talk about praying for a miracle? What happens to the baby?*

So I pick up the manuscript thinking maybe I'll read the first page or two, but I read through the first chapter. It's short. I like that – and I think most readers do as well. So I find myself reading the second chapter and the third. The writer seems to have a flair for the dramatic. The story is suspenseful. This is good. It'll keep the reader turning the pages, anxious to learn what the next chapter holds.

By now, I'm developing an empathy for the writer and the situation in which he finds himself. This empathy creeps up on me, and before I know it I'm pulling for the guy and his wife and their unborn child.

Two hours go by, and I'm still reading.

Now, book publishers are in the business of making decisions to publish or to pass on manuscripts that are brought to their attention. These decisions don't always come easily. But when you're a publisher, and your mind is tired from editing all day, and you find yourself captivated by a story and staying up reading till nearly midnight, it's a sign...

– *Trent Angers, S.F.O.*
Editor & Publisher

For Ephraim

Acknowledgements

I would first like to thank God – the giver of all gifts and the source of all light and love – for His grace during this time of trial in my family's life. I thank my wife, Ashley, whose patience, love and compassion as a mother challenge me every day to be a better father. I am grateful to my parents, Larry and Peggy Judice, and my in-laws, Randy and Ann Guillotte, who gave us their unwavering support while I was writing this book.

A special thanks to Ed Boustany and Sandy Hindelang for the time they spent away from their families in their endless efforts to help spread this message of faith, hope, and the power of prayer. I owe a debt of gratitude to Trent Angers and the staff at Acadian House Publishing for their dedication to this project and their passion in helping to make it a reality.

Thanks to Father Joe Breaux and the men who sat around his table discussing the meaning of Christian manhood and supporting one another in countless ways. The spiritual formation and encouragement I received there prepared me to face the challenges that lay ahead.

I will never forget the role my friend John Listi played in this story. Besides my wife, he was my closest companion on this journey and became my rock at St. Thomas More High School. I was encouraged to write this book by my former teacher and now colleague, Mary Collins, to whom I will be forever grateful.

Lastly, and most emphatically, I would like to thank the entire St. Thomas More school community for being the hands and feet of Christ and for exemplifying what it means to be "seekers of truth, individuals of character, and God's servants first." Your prayers did not go unanswered.

– C.J.

Contents

WAITING
FOR
ELI

Chapter 1

A question for the ages

I WAS LOOKING OUT OF A WINDOW IN THE back of my classroom in the spring of 2005 as the school year was coming to a close. I was feeling more than just a little nostalgia and sadness, because I would be leaving the teaching job and the people I had been with for four years.

During that time, I had taught social studies to seventh and eighth graders at Cathedral-Carmel, a Catholic school in Lafayette, Louisiana. In just two days, my job here would end and I'd be moving on to St. Thomas More, a Catholic high school across town.

Though I was sad to be leaving the Cathedral-Carmel school community – and the people I'd grown fond of over the years – I was equally excited about the new job, the new adventure in teaching.

And, so was my wife, Ashley, who worked as a neonatal nurse at Women's & Children's Hospital in Lafayette. In fact, her place of employment and my new workplace would be just a few blocks from one another. We had a six-months-old son, Ephraim, and we were considering having another child. The higher pay at the new job would come in handy if our family were to grow.

As my days at Cathedral-Carmel were winding down, in the last day or two, I was running my classes in a more relaxed, less structured manner, as many teachers do when the end of school is upon us. For one thing, I gave my students in each class an opportunity to ask me any personal question they wanted. I, of course, reserved the option to answer it or not.

A hand went up, and a male eighth grader asked a question that caught me off guard.

"Coach Judice, what is your greatest fear?"

I had to stop and think for a minute. I had never been asked that question before.

"My greatest fear would be to have a child with a mental or physical handicap," I responded.

I answered in that manner because, as an admitted perfectionist, I didn't think I could handle having a handicapped child. There would be too many responsibilities that would be out of the ordinary, non-routine; it would require patience and parenting skills I did not possess. I'm a very methodical and disciplined person. I'd go as far as to say I am obsessive when it comes to following routines; I have trouble coping with situations I cannot control. (There's a lot to be said for keeping things in order, you know.)

* * *

My first three years at my new teaching job were enjoyable and gratifying. I made numerous new friendships with coworkers and gained the respect of many of my students. I entered this new place of employment with certain career expectations: to eventually be a head assistant basketball coach and to teach American history.

As I finished my second season on the basketball court, I realized I was missing a lot of time with my son Ephraim and decided to walk away from coaching. However, I still had a desire to be involved in school activities, and I was considering campus ministry.

I had gotten to know and like the head of the campus ministry program, John Listi. I felt connected to him the first time I met him. We became friends and weight-lifting partners. His job included conducting various retreats and other activities designed to deepen and enrich the religious and spiritual lives of the students.

John and I forged a bond rather quickly. He asked me if I would be willing to help with campus ministry. I had always had a personal relationship with God, though I was the only one who knew about it. For most of my life, religion was a personal thing. I bought in to the old adage: The two things one should never discuss in polite company are religion and politics. But my attitude on this subject was about to change.

After joining the campus ministry team, I was invited by a priest named Father Joe Breaux to attend regular suppers with other young men for fellowship and personal growth in our relationships with God. The men who sat around this table had a lot in common: We all taught at St. Thomas More, we were all married with children, and we all wanted to help to redefine the role of manhood that we felt society had so badly distorted. We actually ministered to each other, reinforcing one another's beliefs and attitudes. We hoped to serve as good role models of Christian manhood for the students at our school.

The months I spent in fellowship with these men toughened me up and prepared me for the biggest challenge of my life, a challenge I would have to face in the not-too-distant future.

*   *   *

Well before the conception of our second child, Ashley and I discussed at length whether we were ready to increase the size of our family. The central issue was whether we could handle it financially,

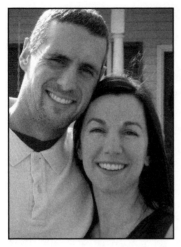

*My wife Ashley and I pose
for a picture in December
2009. We've been through a
lot together and have drawn
upon one another's strengths
since we were married in
2001.*

emotionally, logistically. She was clearly in favor of
the idea well before I was. Ashley usually gets to
decisions faster than I do. I tend to think things
through very thoroughly, sometimes over-thinking
them. Some would say I obsess over things.

I also prayed for guidance – a lot. I prayed and
asked God to show me the way, to help me make
the right decisions. On a retreat in the fall of 2007,
I asked for the peace and grace necessary to surrender control over the situation to Him – to submit
to His will, not mine.

Ashley and I talked a lot about when we wanted
the baby to be born, so we could plan for her mater-
nity leave. I had the idea in my head that we could
control this and a lot more involving our second
child. Looking back on it now, I'm sure God must

have been quite amused at my attitude, at my illusion that Ashley and I were the ones in control.

After all was said and done, we were expecting a baby in February of 2009 – and we were very excited about it. Thus, I began my eighth year of teaching on a high. Life seemed perfect.

My friend John Listi had approached me about being a speaker at a religious retreat, one we refer to as *Kairos*, a Greek word meaning "on God's time." The retreat is offered to junior and senior students who want to re-examine their relationship with God and try to strengthen it. The students who attend get to hear the personal testimony of some of their peers, as well as that of a chosen faculty member, who speaks about how his relationship with God has changed his life.

My presentation was to be a personal testimony about how God had gradually become a larger and larger influence in my life. I worked hard to prepare the presentation and was approaching that weekend with unusual anticipation. As the last week of September rolled around, I was expecting that week to be the best of my life. My wife had reminded me that we had an appointment soon for a routine ultrasound, which would provide a picture of our baby in the womb.

I was so alive! I was going to find out if we were going to have a girl or another boy, and I was going to begin my campus ministry by making possibly the most important presentation of my life. Life just didn't get any better than that. These are the thoughts I had as I drove to meet my wife at the doctor's office.

When I arrived we sat in the waiting room for a while and then they brought us in to do the ultrasound. When it began, we anxiously asked the ultrasound tech not to tell us what sex the baby was until we knew the baby was okay. The tech looked perplexed as she worked with the machine. I could tell by the look on my wife's face that something was wrong. Being a neonatal intensive care nurse, she sees babies with problems every day in her line of work.

"Everything is okay, right?" I said to the ultrasound tech.

She hesitated to answer as she continued to struggle with the machine.

"I'm just having a little trouble finding some measurements for his brain," she responded.

I felt a little sick to my stomach when she said that. Hoping to get some reassurance from Ashley that this was something typical in a routine ultrasound, I looked over at Ashley and saw fear in her eyes. The tech quietly walked out of the room.

Tears began welling up in Ashley's eyes.

"I knew something was wrong. I really thought when we got here today we were going to find out the baby did not have a heartbeat," she said. "I was so nervous in the waiting room before you got here, and I didn't know why."

I stood there not knowing what to say as I tried to absorb what I was seeing and hearing.

It seemed like an eternity before a second tech walked in. As she entered I noticed she looked more experienced, and I felt a little stressed. I expected her to say that the first tech was less experienced and had made a rookie mistake. But instead, she blurted out:

"You are going to have a boy. Congratulations."

She then proceeded to try to get the same measurements that the first tech was trying for, but with no success.

"We're going to bring you guys to another room. The doctor will be with you shortly," she said.

Anxiously, we began waiting for the doctor. When she arrived she informed us that she could not locate part of our son's brain, his cerebellum. She told us she was referring us to a specialist, and that we should meet with the specialist the next day.

Ashley began to cry, and because of my ignorance and shock I didn't know what to say or do.

As I walked out of the office with my wife, that moment at Cathedral-Carmel four years earlier replayed in my mind:

"Hey, Coach, what is your greatest fear?"

My greatest fear was to have a mentally or physically handicapped child. And in the blink of an eye, it had become my reality.

Chapter 2

Aftershock

I COULD BARELY HOLD MY CELL PHONE in my hand as I tried to dial my friend John Listi at St. Thomas More High School. His voice mail answered and, after the routine voice message played and a beep followed, I tried to speak. I started to ask him to pray with the group of students with whom he would be assembled that night at school, but my voice broke and I could not even get the words out of my mouth.

My wife and I drove home from the doctor's office in two different vehicles because we had gone in separate cars. I normally listen to music or talk radio, but I drove home in silence and disbelief, staring off into space the entire time.

We arrived home almost simultaneously. We

didn't really know what was wrong with our son. I sat in the living room of my home and started to cry. I was experiencing a psychological pain so great that I couldn't hold myself up, or focus on anything that would give me any sort of comfort.

My mind raced with questions as the situation we were faced with settled in. Would we have a baby with just half a brain? What kind of life would that be for any human being?

In desperation, I picked up my cell phone and dialed Father Joe's number. He had become like a second father to me, and I needed to talk to someone. I knew if I could find comfort from someone it would be from him. He answered his phone, and as I tried to tell him I needed help I began to cry again. He could barely understand what I was saying.

"Do you need me to come over?" he asked.

"Yes," I replied.

Within fifteen minutes he was at our home. When he walked through the door, I hugged him and wept in his arms.

"Father, something is wrong with my son," I said.

I sat on the couch in my living room, and Father rubbed my back as he asked about my immediate thoughts and concerns. I responded by saying I was scared. That is a feeling I had rarely experienced in my life. Fear of the unknown will test one's faith beyond description.

How would this affect my marriage?

How would it affect my relationship with my older son?

Would this destroy our financial ability to pay for our children's planned Catholic education?

My in-laws, Randy and Ann Guillotte, showed up just as Father Joe was leaving. Randy thanked him for coming and told him that he appreciated his ministering to us in our time of need. I shook my father-in-law's hand very firmly – a sign of mutual respect and understanding between men – and then as our eyes met I bent over in tears. In my moment of weakness we bonded in a way I don't think we had ever bonded before.

"I know, bud. No matter what it takes, we'll take it on," he said in a calm voice.

Just the realization that Ashley and I were not alone was a great comfort to us.

My parents, Larry and Peggy Judice, arrived shortly after my in-laws. They had come to drop off our son, Ephraim. We tried our best to hide from Ephraim the fact we were devastated. We acted as though everything was fine. After putting him to bed, we tried to get some sleep. It was a surreal feeling as we turned out the lights that night. We were lying next to each other but our minds were a million miles away.

The next day, Ashley wasn't scheduled to work, so she stayed home. Her mom came over to provide comfort and support. They talked about what would be a good name for the new baby, and they also spent a little time shopping, to try to get Ashley's mind off of our unborn son. Still, Ashley was anxious as she anticipated the afternoon appointment with the specialist to whom we had been referred.

Though I thought about staying home from work that day, I just couldn't. I thought the best way I could serve my family was by doing my job. I also believed being around the students and doing something I loved would uplift me. I figured I could announce to my students that I was going to have another son, but that I knew there was something terribly wrong with him. When we prayed before the start of each class, I would ask them to pray for him. I was hoping to get through the day without breaking down in front of my students. I thought if they saw that side of me I would lose all effectiveness in the classroom.

My first two classes went pretty well, and I managed to hold my composure. My sophomores were very compassionate, and I expected that from them. As lunch approached, I was wondering how I would address my juniors that afternoon.

At lunch time my principal approached me to ask about my son. He had not seen me during the day up until that point and said he wanted me to know that the entire community was praying for us and was there to support us. He said he was surprised I had come to work. He had spoken to Father Joe the night before, and expected that I would stay home. I told him I would rather be here with my students than sitting at home thinking about it. As the bell rang to end the lunch period I was dreading having to teach the next class.

My fifth-hour class was the roughest group I had that year, a class full of tough guys. Many of them reminded me of me in high school. They were on the verge of manhood and were searching for what manhood is all about. If there was one class in which I did not want to lose my composure, this one was it. If I did, there was no way I could keep them on task.

On any given day when this class prayed, I might get a mumbled Hail Mary or Our Father out of them. So before I began to lead prayer that day I didn't expect much of a difference – even after I would inform them about my son. As they rose to pray I looked all of them squarely in the eyes and tried to tell them the same thing I told my previous classes. I felt my emotions rising.

"I found out yesterday that I am going to have another son, but I also found out that there is something terribly wrong with him. I don't know what your faith life is like, but right now faith is all I've got," I said.

I then bowed my head and tried to start praying, but instead I broke down and began to cry. There was silence for what seemed like a long time.

And then it happened.

One of my female students began to say the Our Father. As I sat there overwhelmed with grief, all of them began to pray. They prayed so loud and so clearly I could barely believe it. It was beautiful.

Was this the same class who had prayed with such seeming apathy all year?

I have been teaching for eight years and I may teach another forty; but I don't think I will ever have a moment quite like this again. It was obvious to me even then: My unborn son was already making his mark.

That afternoon I met my wife at the doctor's office. We sat in the waiting room and chattered nervously. We were escorted into the examination room and greeted by her. She examined my wife using a new, advanced ultrasound machine. She immediately located the baby's head, which on this machine looked more lemon-shaped than oval-shaped. She explained that she had examined the pictures from the original ultrasound and had located a small opening in our son's spinal cord. This neural tube defect could cause the entire brain to be out of place. This explained why we could not find my son's cerebellum in the initial ultrasound. The doctor said our son had water on his brain, a condition called hydrocephalus, which could be an indicator of spina bifida. She expressed her deepest sympathy to have to inform us of this – then she proceeded to ask my wife if she wanted to terminate the pregnancy. Somewhat shocked by this question, Ashley recoiled and looked her in the eyes.

"That is not an option," she said resolutely.

"I apologize if I offended you, but it's my job. I have to ask," the doctor said.

She then told us she would like to monitor Ashley for the rest of the pregnancy and would get us some information on spina bifida. Prior to our leaving, she asked one of her nurses to draw some blood from Ashley. She said a blood test would confirm an elevated level of protein, and that this was a routine test taken to confirm spina bifida in a fetus still in the womb.

That night, Ashley and I sat alone as she examined the information given to her by the doctor. I sat quietly across the room from her, trying to do some school work. Ashley started to cry as she began to read some statistics out loud. Eighty percent of couples who find out their child has a neural tube defect choose abortion. Seventy-five percent of babies with neural tube defects are miscarried before twenty weeks of pregnancy. A child with severe hydrocephalus may have several learning disabilities and, depending on the degree of the neural tube defect, could be paralyzed from the waist down. His sexual organs could possibly never function properly, and he may never have control of his bowel movements.

Ashley looked at me through tear-filled eyes in this moment of human weakness.

"I'm going to hell. I am actually thinking about aborting this child," she said.

I stood up, held her by the shoulders and looked her in the eye.

"This is not your fault. It's not my fault. It just happened. God has a purpose for this child, and He has given him to us. We must trust in Him the way Ephraim trusts in us," I said.

I just knew if we trusted in God the way a child trusts in his or her parent, everything would be okay. I just knew it.

We had thrown around a few names for either a boy or a girl, but had not yet decided on a specific one. We wanted something unique. Because we had spent so much time deciding on our first son's name, we didn't want our second son to be short-changed. Our oldest son's name was biblical, and we wanted a biblical name for our unborn son as well. Ashley wanted to call him Eli. I was okay with that, but I wanted a more solid biblical name, so I suggested Elijah.

We agreed on Elijah Paul Judice.

Now, when we prayed for him, everyone around us would know him by name.

Chapter 3

It would take a miracle

OCTOBER 2, 2008, WAS THE FIRST DAY of the rest of my life.

After being hit with the devastating news the night before and examining the potential outcome of what my unborn son's life could be, I attempted to maintain some sense of normalcy in my everyday routine. That morning at the gym, I saw that the regular crowd was there, and they could tell by the look on my face that something was really wrong. As they asked me questions I was not prepared to answer, I began to feel a sense of hopelessness. When a guy finds himself in a predicament such as mine it is easy to want to withdraw from the world and just disappear. Fear can have a paralyzing grip on a person's life, and I must admit I was nearly paralyzed by fear myself.

Thursday is the day we celebrate weekly Mass at our school, and after first period I headed for Mass with a heavy heart. As teachers we are asked to sit among our students during Mass, but I found a place on a bench away from my class where I could keep an eye on them. As the priest – Father Howard Blessing, a pastor of one of the local parishes – walked toward the altar during the entrance hymn, I found myself singing louder than ever before.

As Father Blessing rose to proclaim the Gospel, I began to feel an eager anticipation to hear what would be read on this particular day. He said it came from the Gospel of Matthew:

> *(Jesus) called a little child and had him stand among them. And he said, "I tell you the truth, unless you change and become like children you will never enter the kingdom of heaven. Therefore, whoever humbles himself like this child is the greatest in the kingdom of heaven. And whoever welcomes a little child like this in my name welcomes me."*

When I heard this passage, I felt like God was speaking directly to me. These were the same words I had referenced the night before when talking with my wife, Ashley. I felt God was acknowledging the fact that Ashley and I had turned to Him in hope and prayer and not to the darkness in despair. I imagined Him saying to me: "Fear not the world, for I have conquered it, and with that conquered your fear. Have faith in me and I will deliver you." In that moment, God seemed to be offering a choice and a once-in-a-lifetime opportunity. He seemed to be saying, "Surrender your will to me, and I will give you rest."

I guess I could have chosen to face this alone, but instead I chose to let Him carry me. At that moment I knew for the first time ever that I was not in control of the events in my life. I had spent thirty years on this earth thinking I was the one in control. And within the span of twenty-four hours that illusion was shattered. I had tried to dictate my life on my terms, but now I felt compelled to surrender to the will of God and to begin to try to understand His will, not mine.

Following Mass we always have a series of announcements before we return to class to complete the rest of the school day. My friend John Listi, who leads music ministry at each Mass, walked up to me and hugged me.

"Man, we were singing so loud and hard for you up there. How are you?" he said.

I then proceeded to tell him about the event that had occurred the night before and how I felt God was speaking to me through the Gospel that day.

"Can I tell them?" he asked.

"Yes," I said.

"I'll be right back," he said.

Just before our principal could take the microphone to send the students to second period, John jumped in front of him. What happened next is something I will never forget for the rest of my life. John stood before twelve hundred students, faculty, staff and parents with tears in his eyes and addressed them.

"I want twelve hundred hearts... right now to pray with me for a miracle for Elijah Paul Judice, the unborn son of Chad and Ashley Judice, who has been diagnosed with spina bifida.

"We pray, heavenly Father, that you may heal this child. Chad and Ashley, we admire your courage, we are behind you, and we love you."

John left the podium, we walked toward each other, and we hugged again. I know it was one of the most powerful things these students had ever witnessed. I could feel it.

*   *   *

Several weeks earlier – before we got the shocking news about our unborn son – I had committed to attend a three-day *Kairos* retreat that would be starting in just a few days.

However, I was thinking about skipping the retreat and staying home because it had been a tough week for Ashley and me. But Ashley urged me to go. She said she couldn't think of a better place for me to be than in a state of prayer.

So I spent the weekend with about fifty students, the largest number ever to attend a *Kairos* retreat put on by St. Thomas More. In fact, some of the participants were not even students from our school; fifteen had come from another Catholic high school to observe how to put on a retreat like this.

Upon arrival at the retreat site, I placed my bags in my room and went to meet the rest of the group in the general meeting hall. I was to be the first speaker in a series of talks. We made a large circle, and each student and adult leader was asked to introduce himself to the group and state why he chose to attend the retreat.

Right before I was to give my testimony, Father Joe called me aside and spoke to me.

"This is your moment. Be naked up there, and let them see who God made you to be," he said as he looked me in the eye.

I was fired up when I took the floor, and I got right to the point.

"My name is Coach Judice, and I came here this weekend to ask you to pray with me for a miracle," I said as I fought back the tears and emotions that rose up from deep inside of me.

I gave my testimony, which described how my relationship with God had grown through the ups and downs of my adolescent and college life into adulthood. I concluded with a detailed explanation of my son's condition and explained that my greatest fear had become my reality. I told them I was handling it with God's help and that I had surrendered my will to Him.

After my talk, my friend John Listi told me he had never seen the students so enthralled and so into a retreat.

The weekend turned out to be phenomenal for me. It was an even better experience than the first time I had attended. In fact, it was very healing for me to be able to express my innermost thoughts and feelings with the participants. We prayed all weekend for Eli and for his miraculous healing.

I returned home Monday night with a refreshed spirit and a firm commitment to pray daily for my unborn son, his brother and my wife. My earnest prayer for my family would continue the next day at school. And it has never ended.

Chapter 4

The mountain is moving

B EFORE LEAVING FOR CLASS ON THE
Tuesday after the *Kairos* retreat, I asked Ashley
if she would meet me at school during second hour
to pray with me on my break. I waited for her in
the library, and when she arrived we proceeded to
the chapel.

Upon entering the chapel we were met by John
Listi and a young man who had attended *Kairos*
that weekend. I asked them to join us in prayer for
Eli. Also, two women were praying in the chapel,
mothers of students attending St. Thomas More. I
did not realize it at the time, but parents are always
praying in the chapel, throughout the day. They
pray for the students and the entire school community. We told them what we were praying for, and

they agreed to join us.

Ashley sat in a chair next to me as I kneeled in front of the Blessed Sacrament and began to pray a series of prayer cards. After completing them, I tried to pray out loud straight from my heart. I asked the Virgin Mary to intercede on our behalf, to ask the Lord, her son, to heal my son. I couldn't stand the thought of my son suffering. I could barely speak and began sobbing.

With every tear that ran down my face, I could feel the healing beginning to take place inside of me. I could feel the strength of my wife as she held my hand and prayed with me.

Following our time in the chapel, Ashley and I returned to the library to read a couple of letters I'd received from students who attended the weekend retreat. I read the letters aloud, and it was clear to both of us that the students had gotten a lot out of the retreat – and were moved by Eli's story.

Coach Judice:

My name is Jacob Nelson, from Catholic High.... The first day when you gave us your testimony, I fought back tears.... What really got me was what you said about your unborn son, Eli. The strength and faith you and your wife must have blows me away. I pray and wish that I can have the courage, strength, and faith in God that you do....

Just to let you know, I will pray for you, your family and Eli every day until I hear about how great he is doing. He will receive many prayers as I dedicate several rosaries to him....

God bless. Stay strong...

When I finished reading the letter and looked at my wife, she had tears in her eyes.

"This is a miracle. I went to a retreat and prayed with students for a miracle. God has given us one," I said, referring to the way that Eli's story had moved this student's heart.

This was the first clear-cut, concrete evidence of the impact that Eli's story would have on the school community.

I knew it would be a long walk from October to February, but I was willing to make that walk with God's help. I had already determined that I could not do this alone. I was rededicating my life to prayer. I could not control the outcome of Eli's condition, but I could control how I chose to handle the situation each and every day.

My life would become a constant prayer – and in this would be my strength. All the questions and uncertainties that swirled in my head had to do with future events over which I now realized I had no control. So, in a very real sense, for the first time in my life I truly "let go and let God."

To give me a boost in morale and a push in the right direction, John Listi sent me an e-mail that afternoon. I read it before leaving school.

Chad,

... Most people would be caving under this and cursing God. Instead you are clinging to Him and leading others to do the same. Amazing! Little Eli is already a messenger for God. He has called everyone to believe in God's miraculous love, and everyone is responding.

Kids who have never prayed in class before are praying for Eli. Parents are hearing these cries and are praying again for their children and loving them unconditionally like they should. And young men are seeing a man of God go to war for his family right before their eyes. They heard you ask God to spare Eli and afflict you instead. That is true fatherly love.... You and I have no real idea how powerfully the Holy Spirit is working through you, Ashley, Ephraim and Elijah right now.... God is so good.

Hang in there, my brother. We are all with you.
– John

Unbelievable things began to unfold for Ashley and me the very moment we said "yes" to God and chose life for our unborn son. We stared the unknown in the face and trusted in our Creator.

Wednesday, October 8, 2008, was a big day for Ashley and me. This is the day we were to get the results of the blood test ordered by the doctor the previous week.

The hours passed slowly throughout the school day as I anxiously waited for a phone call to hear the results. By the end of seventh period, I had not received that call. I began to think that maybe I would have to wait another day before getting the test results.

I had placed the phone face-down on my desk, and before packing my bags and preparing to leave for the day I picked it up and flipped it over. Then I saw a text message:

"Got blood work back, it was normal! – Ashley."

I immediately dialed Ashley's number and asked her what explanation the doctor gave her for the test results. I distinctly remembered the doctor saying the test would show an elevated protein level, that all mothers carrying a fetus with a neural tube defect get that result. Ashley relayed the doctor's exact words:

"I don't know how to explain this, but your protein levels are normal. I am not sure what is going on, but congratulations."

This is the first piece of good news on the medical front that we had heard since the diagnosis. The good doctor may not have had an explanation, but that didn't matter to me. I didn't need one. I knew what was happening. I had just spent the previous weekend with a group of teenagers trying to discover God in their lives and praying in unison for the healing of my son.

The miracle we had prayed for was beginning to happen.

I arrived on campus early the following morning. It had been roughly a week since I announced my son's condition to the school community. I knew the situation was still fresh in everyone's mind. As the bell rang for the school to assemble for Mass that morning, I felt compelled to say something to the entire school community before Mass started. After all of the students had filed in and one of our administrators was about to settle them down, I asked him a favor.

He asked the students to quiet their hearts and minds for Mass, then he introduced me and allowed me to say a few words. I had not written this down or even really thought it through, but I proceeded to walk up to the podium. When I looked out over the twelve hundred people staring back at me, I took a deep breath and began to speak.

"I just wanted to take this opportunity to thank the student body, faculty, staff and parents for all of the prayers you have said for my family and me this past week. I know I could never have made it through the worst week of my life without them. I spent the past weekend on a retreat with some of you, and we asked God for a miracle. Since I have returned home I have seen two. I have seen an unborn child bring teenagers to prayer and to Jesus Christ. That's miracle number one.

"Yesterday, my wife received the results of an initial blood test. Every mother carrying a child with a neural tube defect is supposed to receive a test with an elevated protein level. My wife's test came back normal. The doctor cannot explain it. We don't need an explanation. I know what is happening. That's miracle number two.

"I stand before you as a witness to the power of prayer and the love of God the Father and his son, Jesus Christ. Whether you know it or not, He lives in you. Jesus said if you have faith the size of a mustard seed you can move a mountain. Well, the mountain is moving. Keep praying. He hears you."

Area of Louisiana where Eli's story unfolds

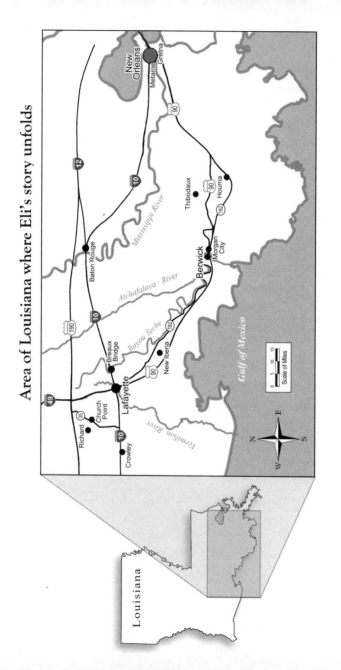

Louisiana

Chapter 5

A visit with the healing priest

THE AFTERNOON AFTER I ADDRESSED the school community at Mass, I was in a big rush to leave school and meet my wife. We were going to Berwick, a town about seventy miles east of Lafayette, to meet with a priest, Fr. Manny Fernandez.

Now, Fr. Manny is no ordinary priest. He is a healing priest. We were fortunate to get an appointment with him, especially on short notice.

Father Manny is one of several children born to a poor family in the Philippine Islands. He felt called to the priesthood at a young age. He entered the seminary as a teenager, with the help of outside funding. After he was ordained, he became a missionary and was assigned to mission work in Africa.

While there, he contracted a disease from one of the people he was treating and became extremely ill. He was declared clinically dead after suffering with the disease for a while, only to awaken the following day completely healed. He was then sent home to his family in the Philippines, and after recovering was told by his superiors that he was not physically able to serve as a missionary. Depressed, he remained in the Philippines and prayed for guidance. Someone in his family became deathly ill, and Fr. Manny was asked to pray over her. Describing a burning sensation in his hands as he prayed over her, he said he could feel the Holy Spirit moving through him to her. A day later she arose from her sick bed, completely healed.

Fr. Manny then left the Philippines and made his way to the United States and ended up in Breaux Bridge, a small town just a few miles east of Lafayette. He was taken in by a couple there as he began his priestly ministry in the Catholic Diocese of Lafayette. He eventually became the pastor of St. Stephen Church in Berwick.

Word of his gift of healing traveled fast. Many have witnessed his ability to call on the power of the Holy Spirit to heal people when medical treatment didn't work.

Ashley and I were blessed to have the opportunity to meet him.

We were determined to get to Berwick before

5:30 that evening to attend the Mass he would be saying. Our plan was to go to Mass and then meet with him one on one afterward.

From the outside, the church looked much smaller than it actually was. The inside was beautiful. The altar was surrounded by the nativity scene, and there was a statue of Mary holding the crucified Christ next to the priest's chair.

Several women were praying the rosary, and Ashley and I joined in. There wasn't much of a crowd in church that day, but Fr. Manny proceeded with the celebration of the Mass anyway. The gospel he read was from the writings of Matthew.

Ask and it will be given to you; seek and you shall find; knock and the door will be opened to you.

This gospel message was so appropriate for our particular situation that it seemed that God was speaking directly to us. He was inviting us to reach out in faith and ask for His help – just ask.

I will never forget what happened that night after Mass in Fr. Manny's home as we visited and he prayed for us.

Father greeted us as we walked into his office in the rectory. We sat on the couch opposite him, and he began to ask us a few questions about Eli. Ashley explained our medical situation and told him about our older son, Ephraim.

"Do you go to church every Sunday? Do you

bring your older son?" he asked.

Ashley told him that we did both. Then he asked us something we had not been asked in our seven years of marriage:

"Do you pray together?"

We were stumped. I knew that we prayed individually, but at that moment I realized that we seldom prayed together as a couple, except during Mass.

"God has allowed this to happen for a reason. He wants you to pray together, as a family," Fr. Manny said.

I had never met this man before that evening, but I felt he was delivering a message from God Himself.

Fr. Manny said he wanted to bless us and pray over us, then he asked if we wanted to go to confession. He said it would be good to go to confession so we could pray with pure hearts. We agreed to go. He asked me to go and sit in another room while he heard Ashley's confession.

As I was waiting for him and looking at some pictures in an album, I could tell he had a strong connection with his parishioners and others with whom he came in contact. When I looked up from the album, he was standing next to me.

"Are you ready?" he asked.

"Yes," I answered.

He began walking in a small semicircle around

me and called upon the Holy Spirit.

"Come, Holy Spirit, beloved of my soul. I adore you. Enlighten me, guide me, strengthen me, consol me. Tell me what I should do. Give me your orders. I promise to submit myself to all that you desire of me, and accept all you permit to happen to me. Let me only know your will."

He then sat next to me and heard my confession. When I was finished he told me to close my eyes. He began praying over me, and his thumb touched my head, and I felt a peace I had never felt in my life. I felt like I was floating. I felt the Holy Spirit, and I knew it. When we finished Fr. Manny took me into the room to meet Ashley.

We sat in the office together and he began to give us some specific instructions. He had a bottle of St. Joseph's healing oil in his hands. He anointed both of our foreheads, our hands, and Ashley's belly. He told us that every night from now until Eli's birth we should do the same thing. We should also anoint Ephraim and have him pray with us. Because he is a child, it would be good to have him pray with us, for God will hear his prayer most certainly because of his innocence. Fr. Manny then told us to recite the prayer to the Holy Spirit. He directed me to anoint Ashley's belly three times, making the sign of the cross, and say the following:

"By the oil of St. Joseph, Lord, please heal Eli's spina bifida and the hydrocephalus on his brain.

May he be born healthy."

Then we should say one Our Father, one Hail Mary, and one Glory Be, he added.

Ashley and I promised to begin praying together and to follow his instructions. Then Fr. Manny began to pray over us. I could remember how much our older son moved in his mom's womb just before he was born. One is not supposed to be able to feel a seventeen-week-old baby in a woman's womb, for the baby is about the size of a small hand at this stage. Father began to pray over Ashley, and as we placed our hands on her belly I could feel my son moving – just as much as I had when Ashley was nine months pregnant with our first son.

Father moved his hands from over Ashley's head and then moved them over our hands. As his hands rested on ours, they felt like they were on fire, literally. He moved his hands over my head, and as he touched me I could feel the heat that had been coming out of his hands now coming out of mine as I continued to feel my son moving in my wife's womb. When he stopped praying, he looked at me and Ashley and asked:

"How do you feel?"

We were both just kind of sitting there in awe.

"Father, I never felt my older son move that way," I said.

"That's because God was touching Eli," Fr. Manny said.

I sat there in silence, knowing that I had just witnessed a miracle. I could feel the presence of God in that room, and I knew He had just touched my son.

As Father walked us out to our car he told us that if we continued to pray and believe, a miracle would happen. He also said if we did not pray and believe, a miracle would not happen.

"Have faith, and come again," he said to us as I cranked up the car to begin our return trip home.

We stopped to eat at a Wendy's on our way home. I was beginning to feel a new sense of peace about the entire situation. We knew the road ahead was long, but we also knew that God was going to be with us on the journey.

I asked Ashley if she felt the same way I did during confession – whether she experienced that extraordinary sense of well-being, that peace beyond all understanding. She said she did.

But she added something I was not expecting. She told me that when Fr. Manny left her in the room to come hear my confession, she could feel the presence of another person in the room; she could feel that she was not alone.

I believe firmly that Jesus was in that room that night to comfort my wife and me. I believe that He held Eli that night and that he continues to hold him in the palm of His hand.

Chapter 6

Waiting for test results

OUR DRIVE HOME FROM BERWICK WAS peaceful, and after a very hard week and a half we finally had a sense of how we would handle the reality of the medical diagnosis that had so unnerved us. For one thing, Ashley would begin attending weekly prayer meetings with Fr. Manny and would receive his blessing each time. These meetings were held in the town of Breaux Bridge, near Lafayette.

A few days after our visit with Fr. Manny, Ashley's doctor asked us to come to her office so she could try to take another look at our unborn son using an advanced ultrasound machine. It would give her a better idea of the location of the opening in his back and could possibly provide a clear view to see if it was a closed lesion. If it was, this would be the best-case scenario.

So Ashley and I returned for another round of ultrasounds. However, every time the doctor took a look at our unborn son, his back was to my wife's spine. He moved very little and never gave us a clear look at his suspected lesion or its location along the spinal canal.

Frustrated by this, the doctor suggested a test called an amniocentesis, in which a long needle is inserted into the uterus of the pregnant female and a sample of amniotic fluid is drawn out to be tested. Ashley was somewhat apprehensive because the test could cause pre-term labor. Still, we wanted to have a concrete answer about his condition, so Ashley agreed to the test. The test result would indicate whether our son's lesion was open or closed.

Conducting the test was our only option if we wanted a clear answer on his condition. Although the doctor had sent pictures of Eli's ultrasound across the country to other doctors for their opinions, she had not received a definite answer.

With that being the case, Ashley and I thought it was in Eli's best interest if we attended the prayer meeting in Breaux Bridge the night before the test was to be conducted.

We got to Breaux Bridge for the prayer meeting at about 6:30 p.m. The lady of the house, Bonnie Latiolais, asked us if it was our first time there, and we said it was. Then we told her we had met with Fr. Manny the week before.

Now, Bonnie and her husband, Rick, are the ones who had taken in Fr. Manny when he arrived from the Philippines in 1987. Their home is his home in America, whenever he wants to be there. He even has his own room, where he spends time when he's away from his priestly duties in Berwick.

Fr. Manny arrived as the last decade of the rosary was being finished and sprinkled all attendees with holy water as he entered. He began his prayer by calling upon the Holy Spirit, and then proceeded to go to each individual to give him or her a personal blessing. We were seated in the middle of the group, so it took a while for him to get to us. When he did, he recognized us and asked if we had any news on the baby. So we told him about the test to be conducted the next day. He then began to anoint us and pray over us. He moved our heads together, and I began to feel that extraordinary sense of peace I had felt at his house in Berwick. Ashley said she could feel a hand behind her head, to keep it from falling, but there was never anyone standing or sitting behind her.

The day after the prayer service, around noon, Ashley went to take the test. Her mom went with her so I would not have to miss work. I wanted to save my days off for when Eli was born. The doctor told Ashley the test results would be known in three to five days.

I was going to keep praying and trusting in God. We had done that so far, and He had not abandoned us. It was at this point in our journey that I decided to make an effort to dedicate one hour of my school day to prayer in the school's chapel. It is amazing how things in a person's life will change for the better if he commits himself to having a dialogue with God each day.

As we were anxiously waiting for the test results, my thoughts returned to the young man from Catholic High who had attended the *Kairos* retreat and had written me such a moving letter. I felt after receiving such a gift from him I owed him some type of response, and so I wrote him.

Dear Jacob:

I was truly touched by your personal affirmation of me on the Sunday morning following my testimony. I was a little shocked to hear what you said, and it caught me off guard. That is why all I could say was a quick "Thank You."

Upon returning home from Kairos and looking at all of my letters in my mailbag with my wife, we came across yours....

My wife looked at me with tears in her eyes as she finished reading your letter ..., and I said, "I prayed for a miracle this weekend and God has given us one."

I was giving my testimony with the outlook that if it made a difference or changed just one person it would be worth it. Obviously, by the reaction of the other participants, it did; but your response was more personal....

You wrote in your letter to me that you wish you had the courage, strength, and faith in God that I have.... I'm here to tell you, son, you do have it. Every man does. The difference between boys and men is that men choose to dig deep down inside and have the fortitude to act on their convictions.

I teach American history and I always tell my students that there is not much difference between heroes and cowards except one thing: Heroes face their fears head-on instead of running away from them. Both are scared, and both make choices.

Jesus Christ lives in you, and gives all men a choice, so choose wisely. I don't know you personally, but based on the tone of your letter, I'd bet the farm on you making the right choice.

I just wanted to express my gratitude for your willingness to pray for my family and my unborn son. Your prayers and the prayers of many others must be very effective. The Wednesday I returned from Kairos my wife received a blood test result a specialist could not explain. It was normal. A woman carrying a child with spina bifida is supposed to have an elevated protein level. She did not. Since then, she has had to have another test run. My son's case is baffling specialists, and they say they have never seen anything like this. Maybe that miracle we were praying for is happening, and they can't understand it....

As we continued to wait for the test results, Ashley and I had the opportunity to go shopping and spend some quality time together. Since we had discovered our unborn son's condition, we had received a lot of help with Ephraim; he spent quite a bit of time with his grandparents. One of the most difficult parts of our situation was trying to be good parents to our oldest child without constantly over-analyzing the condition of our second. Parenting can be the most physically, emotionally and spiritually exhausting task. But it can also be rewarding beyond explanation. A little time to recharge one's battery is always legitimate. This was the case on that evening, and we had a nice time.

We arrived home a little after eight o'clock. There was a message on the answering machine. The doctor had called and left her personal cell phone number. She said she had the results of the test and asked Ashley to call her.

I saw a pained look on Ashley's face as she tried to keep her composure while speaking with the doctor. Ashley seemed very disappointed in what she was hearing. The news confirmed our worst fear: Our son had an open lesion, and it could continue to get bigger throughout the pregnancy. This would increase his chances of paralysis and loss of bowel control and could mean Eli would be in a wheelchair all his life.

Ashley turned to me with a look of strength and

determination I had never seen in her until that moment.

"We'll keep praying. We'll pray that his lesion remains small," she said.

My faith was renewed by the conviction in her voice. Though modern medicine seemed to be indicating that Eli would never walk, we refused to stop believing that, by the grace of God, our son will walk one day.

Ashley and I cried together as we sat in our house alone. We were down but not out.

Our prayer life was about to go to a new level. And so was God's amazing grace.

Chapter 7

Signs all around me

RECEIVING THE RESULTS OF THE amniocentesis test motivated me to go back to God and ask for help. That hopeless feeling had begun to creep back into my heart after riding high on the news of the original blood test that came back normal.

I got up every day and continued to do my job, continued to be a father to my older son and a husband to my wife, and I began to accept living in a state of unknowing. It's hard to explain this feeling.

The only peace I could muster to continue moving forward was in the hour I spent in prayer every day in the chapel at school. Some days I prayed in fear, other days in frustration and sorrow, and some days in hope.

I never prayed alone. I began making it a habit to ask one of the parents praying in the chapel when I entered to join me. Whether I knew them or taught their child or not, it made me no difference. I just wanted to pray with someone because I believe what Christ said when He told his disciples, "When two or more are gathered in my name, I am there."

One day in late October I went to the chapel to pray, as is my custom. Upon entering the chapel, I saw a blonde-haired woman kneeling before the Blessed Sacrament in prayer. I knelt down next to her, and I asked her if she would be willing to pray with me. Then I introduced myself.

"Oh, my daughter is a freshman and has come home on many nights and told us about your son. I would love to pray with you," she whispered.

We prayed the rosary, then some prayer cards asking for the intercession of the Blessed Mother.

(The term intercession is heard most often among Catholics and some other Christians. It is derived from the words "to intercede," meaning "to act, or advocate, on behalf of another." Thus, intercessors – such as the Blessed Mother and the saints – bring our prayers and petitions to God on our behalf. They serve as go-betweens. The concept is that they have achieved a high level of holiness, that they are closer to God than us mere mortals, and as such communicate with God in ways that we cannot. This is not to imply that God doesn't hear prayers that aren't made through intercessors. An intercessor is essentially an advocate or an ally. Thus, in intercessory prayer, we seek the aid of another to bring our prayers and petitions to God – who alone can work a miracle.)

"Do you have a special relationship with the Blessed Mother?" my prayer partner asked.

I had never been asked that question before, so I hesitated before responding.

"Yes, I guess I do," I answered.

She began to explain in detail about how she had been praying to Mary for years and that Mary was a powerful intercessor. She told me that she felt God has chosen me at this moment in this school for a reason. She believed that God was using my family to show people His power and mercy. She told me she felt that the suffering Ashley and I were enduring was a blessing, a great opportunity to enrich our relationship with God.

I realized that day how blessed we were to be given Eli. Whatever suffering we would endure would be of little consequence on this earth. God was challenging us to live more spiritual lives, to pray more earnestly, and to offer up our sufferings for others.

Eli would become and will always be my stairway to heaven. I have sought a more personal relationship with God in my prayer life each day. And the rewards He has given to us for seeking His grace are many.

As I was leaving for school one morning, Ashley

came to meet me at my car right before I backed out. I quickly stepped on the brake and rolled down the window.

"I just wanted to say that I love you. Here, take this. I know you pray every day, and this is a novena to St. Therese that I just finished. Have a great day," Ashley said to me.

I took the prayer card and put it in the console of the car. I brought Ephraim to school and went on to work, like any other day. I had intentions of bringing the card into the chapel with me, but I forgot it in my car. I did not know it at the time, but Ashley had prayed that prayer card for seven days prior to giving it to me.

A few days later, I was leaving the library after one of my breaks. I had been voicing my concerns about Eli to some of my colleagues. I was telling them that I was frustrated to have to live in the unknown. No matter how much a person loves what he does, or becomes preoccupied with any task, the thought that his child may die in the womb or live a less-than-normal life never leaves his mind. One of my colleagues made a great suggestion, and I adopted it as my new motto.

"Chad, you may not be here tomorrow. Just live one day at a time," she offered.

It was the most sensible advice anyone had given me to that point, and it helped to ground me. I believe God speaks to us every day through different people, and then He gives us the opportunity to realize it. This was just one of many times that this occurred during Ashley's pregnancy.

My phone began to buzz as our conversation was ending. Ashley's voice was on the other end of the line, and she seemed to be in a peculiar mood. She said she was having a really rough day until she got a special delivery.

"I got a rose today," she said happily.

I was surprised and a little embarrassed, because I'm not the one who sent it. I asked her if she knew who did.

"I think it came from my mom. It has a note on it. Do you want to know what it says?"

"Sure."

She then proceeded to read the card: *"Your love is more beautiful than this rose. Love, Eli – Just the way God intended."* Then she told me that when the delivery man dropped off the rose all her colleagues began to cry. Ashley works with some wonderful people at her hospital, and they have proved to be an important source of support for her, just as my colleagues at my job have been for me.

It wasn't until later that night that I realized the significance of that rose. Ashley arrived home with a huge smile on her face and said that St. Therese had sent her the rose as a sign. She said she believed St. Therese had heard her prayer and was interceding for her. She went on to explain that after you say a novena to St. Therese, you ask her to send you a rose – as a sign that your prayers are being heard – then you wait in faith to receive a rose.

I asked Ashley if her mom knew that she had been saying the novena, and she said that her mom had no idea. In fact, when Ashley realized that her mom had sent the rose, she called her. After thanking her mom, she asked what compelled her to send the rose. Her mom replied:

"On my way to work this morning something just told me deep inside you had to have a rose."

Some people would chalk this up to coincidence. Well, I call it our first major God-incidence. He had our attention.

If I needed another sign that Ashley and I were not alone on our journey, I found it a few days later as I was walking down the hall toward my classroom. I noticed a small sticky note on the window of the door to one of the classrooms. I stopped to see what was drawn on the little piece of paper. It was a cross, and in the center of it was a heart. Then my heart fell into my stomach. Inside the heart, clear as day, was the name Eli. Each heart had rays exiting from all sides of the cross, as if Eli's name was giving off a ray of light. I was touched. I continued to walk toward my room and passed another room. That one had a sticker on it, too. I kept walking down the hall, and in utter awe and disbelief, I saw every room had a sticker on it. I eventually realized that every doorway in the entire school had a sticker on it.

Some student or students had taken the time to hand-draw these crosses on sticky notes and proceed to walk the entire school and place one on each doorway. It was to serve as a constant reminder to pray for Eli before each class, each day, until he was born. What a selfless act from a group of people who, because of their age and the world in which they live, might be expected to be more preoccupied with themselves.

I felt God was beginning to reveal something to me that I had not seen before. This was all happening at *this* school, at *this* time, with *these* kids, for a specific reason. I did not understand it, but I knew that day that God was using me and my family.

Eli was no ordinary baby. He had a real purpose that was well beyond my comprehension. In the span of three days I felt God was showing me that this was bigger than just our family, way bigger. It was clear to me that the Holy Spirit was moving

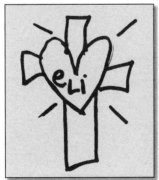

in my life – and in the lives of twelve hundred teenagers at St. Thomas More High School.

Small sticky notes like this one were placed on each door of each classroom at St. Thomas More, a sign that Eli was in the hearts and prayers of the entire school community.

Chapter 8

Hope springs eternal

A S WE ENTERED THE MONTH OF November, I began to feel a sense of hope rather than fear when I prayed. I believe the Lord had spoken directly or indirectly to Ashley and me. We were confident that our prayers were being heard and that they would be answered.

I had begun officiating basketball games every Tuesday and Friday night at local high schools, and my classes were moving along like they did in any other school year. Being preoccupied with my normal routine provided mental breaks from my ever-present concern over Eli's situation.

Each day when I prayed in the chapel, it seemed as though I would meet someone whom I needed to encounter or who needed to encounter me. I remember praying one morning with a mother of one of my students. When I entered the chapel and asked her to pray with me she readily agreed. We did not know each other, but she knew about Eli. When we finished the rosary, she said:

"I did not even want to come to Holy Hour today. God sent you here today to say something to me. I am so glad I came. God bless you and your family. Mine will continue to pray for your son."

That same week, on a Friday, I walked into the chapel to pray and no one was in there. I knelt down and began my rosary. I was praying out loud and was about half way through the third decade when I heard the chapel door open behind me. Since my back was to the door, I could not see who was entering. I heard the ruffling of book sacks and the shuffling of feet as the students from one of the religion classes filed in to take their seats. I heard "Quiet, please" as I continued to pray the rosary aloud.

I recognized the voice. It was Lance Strother, a man who teaches theology and coaches football at our school. He is a graduate of St. Thomas More and is my age, around thirty. He's one of the guys in the fellowship group I meet with monthly at Father Joe's house.

As I started the fourth decade of the rosary I heard his voice and the voices of his students join in. They said the last two decades with me. When we finished the rosary, I continued with another prayer:

"Hail, Holy Queen, we offer up this rosary today and ask that you intercede to our Lord and Savior, Jesus Christ. Ask Him to heal my son Elijah Paul's spina bifida and the hydrocephalus on his brain."

I tried to continue praying, but my voice was cracking and I was overwhelmed with emotion. I began feeling the pain that I had felt the first week I found out about Eli.

"Please heal my son...," I continued.

After a moment of silence, I recited the Serenity Prayer:

> *God grant me the serenity*
> *to accept the things I cannot change;*
> *the courage to change the things I can;*
> *and the wisdom to know the difference.*

When I rose from the kneeler and turned to exit, Lance hugged me. His students sat quietly in their seats, not sure what to think, not sure what to do. Even though I never looked any of them in the eye, I knew it was part of God's plan for them to witness what they had just seen and heard. It was the first time these students had seen a teacher praying like that in front of the Blessed Sacrament. As I was leaving the chapel, I overheard Lance say to his students:

"You thought you were coming in here for a day of reflection and praise and worship. What you saw was a man totally surrender his will to God."

After that day, several of my fellow teachers told me that every day at least one person in their class would pray for me or my family – including students who seldom prayed before.

One day in mid-November, a friend of mine arranged for Ashley and me to contact a couple in Lafayette who had been down the same road we were on. Karen and Peter Fortier had a 25-year-old son named Hunter, and he was born with spina bifida. He lived in Austin, Texas, and was about to graduate from the University of Texas. He was completely self-sufficient and was even dating a young woman very seriously. We could not wait to talk with the Fortiers – people who could truly understand how we felt.

It was a beautiful autumn afternoon, and Ashley and I decided to call them. When Karen answered her phone and I told her who I was, she said she had been expecting my call and was delighted to hear from us. She invited us over for a visit that same day. Ashley and I dropped Ephraim off at my parents' home and then drove to meet the Fortiers at their place.

The Fortiers are two of the most inspiring people Ashley and I have encountered on our journey. As we sat and visited with them that afternoon, we found out some very interesting things. Karen's husband had adopted her two children from her first marriage. The Fortiers badly wanted to have a child of their own, and she eventually became pregnant. She said that during the seventh or eighth month of her pregnancy, she just knew that her son would be born with spina bifida.

When asked how she knew, she explained that she had been helping a group of women put on puppet shows for disabled children around Lafayette. Each puppet had a disability, like the kids in the audience. One day while she was sitting out in the audience watching one of the shows she noticed that one of the puppets was portraying a child with spina bifida. It was an omen, and somehow she knew that instant that her child would be born with this birth defect.

She later asked her doctor about the condition. He told her she was young and healthy and that the chances of that happening were slim to none. Ultrasound technology was not what it is today, so she and her husband did not know for sure about their son, Hunter, until the day he was born. They were devastated. She cautioned us that if we read all the medical information on spina bifida it would do nothing but depress us. Then she added:

"Forget the statistics; your child is not a statistic. He is a person. Only God knows what his limitations will or will not be."

Karen spoke for an hour about the thirty-four surgeries her son underwent and the fact that even though doctors told her he would never walk, she knew he would. After years of physical therapy and determination, her son, with his family's help, not only walks but leads a very normal life. Hearing this brought a new stage of hope to both Ashley and me.

"If you ever need anything, don't hesitate to call," Karen said as we left their home and thanked them again for talking with us.

I have come to believe that God puts certain people in our lives when He wants to teach us things. That day I felt He was saying to us:

"All things are possible through me!"

Karen and Peter Fortier gave us a new way of looking at our situation. Our hope was and is for Eli to be blessed in the way their son has been blessed. Hunter Fortier's story can be Eli's story. And, God willing, it will be.

Chapter 9

A nurse's burden

ONE FRIDAY NIGHT IN NOVEMBER Ashley got home from work looking completely exhausted. It's not uncommon for someone in her line of work to come home like this. She arrives at the hospital at 6:30 in the morning and sometimes does not get home until after 9:00 at night. Her job keeps her on her feet twelve hours a day. Ashley is very reserved when it comes to talking about her work, and when she does open up about it, all she really wants me to do is just listen.

I was so busy trying to get Ephraim ready for bed and the house neatened up that I did not notice how despondent she was that night.

I had made big plans for us for the following evening. I had arranged for my parents to keep Ephraim overnight so Ashley and I could go on a date. We had not had a night to ourselves since we found out about Eli's condition, and I thought our night out alone was much needed at this point. I had made reservations at Ruth's Chris Steak House, one of our favorite places to eat for a special occasion. I could see that Ashley was having a rough month, and I wanted to cheer her up. I thought a dinner and a movie might give us a break from our worries.

As we sat at the table waiting for our food, we talked, but not much. We tried to talk about other things, but the conversation always went back to Eli. I asked her how she was holding up, and I could tell she was fighting back tears as she tried to explain her fears and hopes.

It's hard for someone who works in the medical field to be optimistic. Having faith in the unseen is difficult for someone who sees the worst of the worst every day – especially an expectant mother whose job entails caring for sick babies twelve hours a day.

As we were getting up to leave, I was thinking I would suggest to Ashley that she call Karen Fortier, our new friend with the 25-year-old son with spina bifida. Karen had said any time we needed anything, even if it was just to talk, that we should call her. We were headed for the door when I heard my name being called. I turned around, and who were sitting there but Karen and Peter Fortier. Seeing them and chatting briefly surely lifted our spirits. Maybe it was just a coincidence to run into the very people my wife needed to see. Maybe it wasn't...

We arrived home pretty late after the movie and I saw that Ashley's mood still wasn't much better than it was at supper. So, I finally asked:

"Ashley, what's wrong?"

She began to cry and placed her hand on our son in her belly.

"I lost a baby last night. She died," Ashley said in a sorrowful tone.

Nurses who take care of babies carry a heavy burden when one they are caring for passes away. Then there's the burden of having to inform the parents. My wife had done this on the previous evening before coming home. She wanted to tell me about it, but I was too busy and preoccupied. She explained that the baby was a full-term girl who had been given a clean bill of health and was scheduled to go home that day. But, by early evening a severe medical complication had occurred and the baby eventually died. Ashley held her belly, and in a voice riddled with deep pain and anxiety, she said:

"That baby was normal, and she died. What is going to happen to Eli?"

I sat there and said to her that God had gotten Eli this far and that He had a purpose for him. Our job was to keep trusting. Then I added:

"I have never asked why. Why this happened to

us?"

Then, with tears rolling down my face, I said:

"But I have asked, Why did I not appreciate Ephraim and you the way I should have? Why did this have to happen for me to finally get it, to realize the blessings I have in my life – especially my beautiful wife and healthy child?"

I turned out the light and I held her, and we fell asleep in a matter of minutes, emotionally exhausted.

It seemed that her burden had been lightened somewhat, now that she was able to share her story with me – now that I was listening. Lightening each other's burdens in life is one of the things husbands and wives are supposed to do for one another.

Chapter 10

Praying at Charlene's grave

THE DAY AFTER OUR SUPPER-AND-MOVIE date, Ashley and I attended Mass, then went to join Ephraim and my parents for lunch. After eating, we all piled into the car and rode out into the country to the somewhat famous little community of Richard, about thirty-five miles northwest of Lafayette.

There, we would pray for Eli at the grave of Charlene Richard, whom many in our part of the country refer to as "The Little Cajun Saint."

Charlene Richard was born in 1947 and died of lymphatic cancer at age twelve. She was hospitalized in Lafayette at Our Lady of Lourdes, and was ministered to by a priest named Father Joseph Brennan. He said of her:

"I see Charlene as a witness for people of all ages to the power of resignation and acceptance of God's will. She wasn't different in any way except that when crisis came in her life – and it came early – she accepted it with faith, trust and love."

Though she has not been officially canonized by the Catholic Church, she is thought of by many as a saint because of several documented cases of miraculous cures of people with terminal illnesses; these healings have been attributed to Charlene's intercession.

When we arrived at the gravesite we appeared to be the only people there. Ephraim had fallen asleep, and my dad volunteered to stay in the car with him. My mom came with Ashley and me to the grave. The cemetery is a beautiful place and is extremely peaceful. A picture of Charlene is affixed to her headstone. Kneelers are set up on two sides of the grave, and there is a petition box on top. Ashley and I took a recent picture from an ultrasound, wrote Eli's name on the back, and put it in the box.

Before kneeling to pray, I walked to the headstone, where two accounts of miraculous healings were attached and hanging by a string. These typewritten sheets were laminated to protect them from the elements.

One account was of a father and his daughter who flew to Louisiana from New York to pray at Charlene's grave. The daughter, who had terminal breast cancer, was completely cured, much to the amazement of her physicians. The father, who had lung cancer, found his disease to be in remission when he returned home. The other account was of a woman with colon cancer who prayed at the gravesite and was cured.

Charlene Richard,
'The Little Cajun Saint'

I read both stories to myself, and I knew we had come to the right place.

My mom kneeled facing the headstone and Ashley and I kneeled down on the side of the grave. We began to pray, and as I led the rosary I began to sob. So did my wife and my mother. After completing the last decade I said a prayer to Charlene, asking her to intercede for Eli's well-being. After that, my mom left to check on Ephraim.

It was about forty degrees that day and had been very chilly during our visit. I lowered my head and began to pray silently for peace in my heart. The wind picked up, but instead of the temperature getting colder it got warmer. I felt the rays of the sun on the back of my neck. Then I felt a hand caressing me ever so slightly in the middle of my upper back, as though someone was consoling me.

I opened my eyes, and I looked to my left, thinking it was Ashley. But it wasn't. She was standing at the headstone reading the accounts of the miraculous cures. I kept looking around. Whose hand was it? I was mystified.

We walked over to the church, St. Edward's, and sat in the pews to relax and pray some more. We got settled and I focused on a painting near the altar, and I could barely believe my eyes! There was an image of Abraham being stopped by an angel from sacrificing his son, Isaac. God really had my attention now.

From the start of our ordeal I constantly felt a connection to certain biblical figures, especially Abraham, who was tested by God. Abraham was asked to sacrifice his only son to prove his love for God. Abraham did not want to sacrifice his son, but was obedient to what he understood God's will to be. He trusted in God. In the final moments, God sent an angel to stop him from taking his son's life. Abraham's reward was a covenant with God, who blessed him with as many descendants "as the stars in the sky." I knew from that moment – from the moment I saw this painting, in this church, in this holy place – that Eli was going to be okay.

Ashley and I received a type of healing that day that we had not had up until that point. We grieved at the gravesite but felt a spiritual renewal upon our return. It is an incredible place, and I hope to return one day with my children.

Chapter 11

The baby is kicking

ONE SATURDAY JUST A FEW WEEKS before Christmas, Ashley and I received an unexpected letter that brought tears to our eyes. It was from one of my relatives (a second cousin), Reggie Judice, and his wife, Claire.

Dear Ashley and Chad,

Enclosed is a note from Brother Daniel. I truly feel that your baby is the miracle that Blessed Bro. Arnold needs for canonization. We will keep praying.

Love,
Claire, Reggie, and the boys

In the envelope with this letter was a postcard from a retired Christian Brother who resides in our

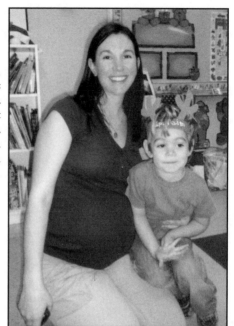

My wife Ashley, seven months pregnant with Eli, enjoys a light moment with our son Ephraim at his school in December 2008.

town. Ashley read it aloud:

> *Dear Claire,*
>
> *We continue to pray for Chad and Ashley and the cure of their unborn child through the intercession of Blessed Arnold, who needs one more miracle for canonization. May you all have a Happy Thanksgiving Day.*
>
> *Brother Daniel*

Claire's father had been very close to the Christian Brothers in Lafayette. Someone in her family had informed Bro. Daniel about Eli's condition. Bro. Daniel began earnestly praying with his fellow Christian Brothers for Eli's healing, and he had informed Claire of their prayers.

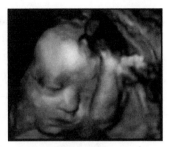

Eli in the womb at 30 weeks

The week after receiving this letter, Ashley had another scheduled ultrasound with the specialist she was seeing. This doctor is a maternal fetal perinatologist, one who specializes in monitoring expectant mothers with high-risk pregnancies, including those with babies diagnosed with spina bifida. Two significant things came out of this appointment.

First, Ashley confirmed that when it was time to give birth to Eli, the delivery would take place in New Orleans. The pediatric neurosurgeon who would perform the procedure worked in a hospital there. My son's pediatrician, who happened to be my godfather, had highly recommended this doctor in New Orleans. Ashley's specialist concurred and would soon begin making plans for us to meet with the doctor who would deliver Eli.

Second, we were delighted by what we saw on the ultrasound. Our son could fully extend his legs, and I saw him literally kick his mom.

Ashley had felt him move on a daily basis, but

at this point in the pregnancy, for him to continue to have that kind of movement was phenomenal. Most children with his diagnosis begin to lose such movement as they get closer to delivery. Eli was due in February, so with a little more than two months left to go, this was great news.

When we returned from the doctor's office, I sent an e-mail to my co-workers, family and friends:

> *Ashley had an ultrasound today. Eli's head looks better, and we saw him move his legs and his toes. This is a positive sign....*
>
> *Two months ago I was contemplating if he would ever walk. Now, when he is a toddler and trying to learn how to walk, I can tell him, "Son, I've seen you do it before, and I know you will do it again."*
>
> *It is a miracle, small but real.*
>
> *The mountain is moving... keep praying... He hears us all.*
>
> *"In the world you will have trouble, but take courage. I have conquered the world." (John 16:33)*

Christmas vacation proved to be the most meaningful one of my life. A two-week break from school would usher in a new year and the fast-approaching birth of our son.

Chapter 12

Manna from heaven

JUST A FEW DAYS BEFORE CHRISTMAS, we received another item in the mail from my cousin Reggie Judice and his wife Claire. It was a Christmas card, and folded inside was a page of hand-written notes about the life of Blessed Brother Arnold, who could be declared a saint one day.

Dear Ashley and Chad,

Enclosed is the information on Blessed Arnold. Please try to keep the Christian Brothers updated on the baby. The Brothers here are informing the Christian Brothers around the world about the wonderful progress that Eli is having.

This tiny baby has brought so many people to God. He is so wonderful, and we have not even been able to meet him yet. Eli is a true blessing.

Love,
Claire and Reggie

I was in awe that the Christian Brothers around the world were praying in unison for our son. They were doing it for a baby and a family in the middle of southwestern Louisiana whom they didn't know and would never meet. I understand they have in the past prayed in earnest for others and that their prayers have been answered.

As I read the information about Bro. Arnold, I was quite amazed as I realized the number of ways that I and my family are connected to him. Bro. Arnold was a member of the order of teaching brothers that founded schools in Europe, the United States and other countries; among the schools they established in southern Louisiana is Cathedral-Carmel in Lafayette – where I was employed as a teacher before going to St. Thomas More.

Bro. Arnold lived in nineteenth century Europe, in the province of Alsace-Lorraine, a region along the border between Germany and France. It just so happens that is the very place my ancestors lived before immigrating to America. During a war between France and Germany in the 1870s he cared for soldiers on both sides who were wounded on the battlefield. In a way, you could say he was a nurse, like my wife. Furthermore, he is remembered for his dedication to prayer to the Holy Spirit, which he believed would strengthen his heart and the hearts of others. I, too, have prayed daily to the Holy Spirit to give me strength in this time of trial. I can conclude only that God had given my family the perfect intercessor in the person of Blessed Brother Arnold. To this day, an image of Bro. Arnold hangs in our home.

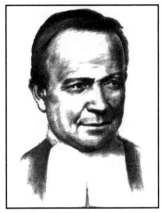

Blessed Brother Arnold

*   *   *

The Mass that evening was the most meaningful Christmas Eve service I ever attended. After communion, the choir sang "Silent Night." In the time of reflection before the closing prayer, I was touched by the presence of the Holy Spirit. The beautiful voice of a young lady singing echoed off the walls of the church. I stared at the crucifix behind the altar, with Ephraim in my arms, and a tear rolled down the side of my face. I realized more profoundly than ever before that the greatest gift I had ever received from God was my wife and children. I knew at that moment I would never be the same again. I had crossed over to the other side; that part of me that had clung to the boyish desires of my past was now gone forever.

Because Ashley had to work at the hospital on Christmas Day, we had to celebrate the holidays with our families over a two-day period. Christmas

Day, Ephraim and I went to my parents', and the following day, when Ashley was off, we went to Ashley's parents' home. This Christmas there was an addition to the guest list. Ashley's parents' neighbor had just lost his wife to cancer a few months earlier. So they invited him over for Christmas dinner.

When we arrived at my in-laws' home my mother-in-law handed me an envelope. It said "Merry Christmas, Ashley and Chad." It was from the next-door neighbor who was going to be joining us for dinner. Ashley opened the envelope and began to cry. She handed me a check that was inside, and I could hardly believe my eyes. It was a check for a substantial amount of money, made payable to cash.

When the generous neighbor arrived a few minutes later, I shook his hand. Our eyes met, and I think we had a glimpse into each other's soul. He could feel my pain for my situation, and I could feel his pain from the loss of his wife.

"Thank you," I said with deep sincerity.

"You are welcome," he responded, as he shook my hand again.

Ashley and her family had hosted a garage sale at the beginning of December to cover the huge cost of hotel rooms that we expected to incur in New Orleans. We were also faced with having to find a place to stay – possibly for a month or two – while Eli remained in the hospital for the necessary surgeries following his birth. While the garage sale raised a portion of the money we would need, we still needed a lot more. So, the check from the kind and thoughtful neighbor was like manna from heaven; it would go a long way toward easing the financial pressure we were under.

The kind neighbor turned to us as we finished dinner, and said:

"I wanted to let you know that I have arranged for you to stay with some friends of mine in Gretna. They are a couple that my wife and I have known for quite some time. In fact, they were some of our best friends. They have a garage apartment behind their home that their daughter used to live in. They said you are welcome to it for as long as you need. It has a bathroom, kitchen and cable television. If you need to wash any clothes, they will assist you with that as well. You have a place to stay and can now take that money and put it on the baby. Their home is located roughly fifteen minutes from the hospital where you will be delivering. When you are discharged, you can stay there until it is time to bring Eli home. Merry Christmas."

As I sat there in amazement I was once again reminded of the importance of trusting in the Lord, trusting that He will provide. The Gospel of Matthew says:

Look at the birds of the air; they do not sow or reap or store away in barns, and yet our Heavenly Father feeds them. Are you not much more valuable than they?... But seek ye first his kingdom and his righteousness, and all things will be given to you as well.

Christmas 2008 was unique for us for a number of reasons. But the most profound reason was that the more we trusted in God the more things in our unstable situation became stable.

With the return of school rapidly approaching and the birth of Eli a little more than a month away, I had a lot for which to be thankful. My hope in God's promise was now turning to confidence in that promise. Every time I thought nothing more amazing could happen, something did.

With my faith at an all-time high and my will to move forward renewed, I couldn't wait to get back to the classroom. I felt that God was just beginning to use me – and the St. Thomas More community – to reveal His omnipotent power.

Chapter 13

Countdown

JANUARY 2009 WAS THE BEGINNING OF the second semester of the school year. Eli was scheduled to be born on February 17, six weeks later. I resolved to step up my prayer time in the chapel in this final stage of preparation for my son's birth.

My daily prayer began to focus more on my first son, Ephraim. I wanted badly to protect him as long as possible from the adverse effects of our predicament. I figured that the person who would be most affected from our stay in New Orleans following Eli's birth would be Ephraim. He would be with my parents, whom he loves very much, but I knew he would miss us, especially Ashley. I was already praying for strength for the time when I would have to leave Ashley and Eli in New Orleans and return home to take care of Ephraim. I dreaded the moment when Ephraim would say, "I want mommy."

I was preparing for the time when I would watch one son suffer physically while having to try to comfort one who would be suffering emotionally. So I put it in God's hands.

One morning in the early part of the month, I went to the chapel and encountered two women with whom I had prayed on several previous occasions. They inquired about Eli's status, then one of them asked me to write an article about our journey with Eli for the next edition of the school newsletter. I readily accepted the invitation.

I figured this would be a good opportunity to collect my thoughts about our bittersweet journey. The piece would be a summary of our experiences and could be used not only as an article but as the basis for a talk.

That weekend, after praying for guidance, I sat at the computer and composed my testimony. It's called "Eli's Witness." (See Appendix 1) I felt then, as I do now, that by the grace of God, when it would be heard it could change people's lives.

My first opportunity to read the testimony would come at a prayer service for Eli, to be held at the school one night just before his scheduled birth. Students, parents and faculty would be invited.

*　　*　　*

February 2, 2009, started out like any other Monday, the beginning of a new week of school. It was just a little more than two weeks from the time Eli was to be born. I was counting the days. I was apprehensive, but hopeful.

Ashley had worked on the previous weekend, so she had the day off and she was coming to school to join me for lunch.

After the bell ending the third period, I made my way to the chapel. When I walked in I recognized a woman who was praying, and we said a rosary together. When we finished, she struck up a conversation.

"You know, I've never met your wife. I'd love to meet her some day," she said.

"Well, you're in luck; she's coming to meet me for lunch within the next five minutes. If you stick around for a few minutes you will get to meet her," I responded.

Just as I finished what I was saying, my cell phone vibrated. It was Ashley calling to tell me she had arrived with our lunch and she wanted me to meet her at the front entrance. When I met her I asked her to accompany me to the chapel. There was someone there I wanted her to meet.

The woman with whom I had been praying greeted Ashley with a big smile.

"It's so nice to finally meet you, Ashley," she said. "I have been praying with your husband for quite a while now. I really believe God is using him and your situation at this school to show these students something pretty incredible. I think your son will touch many people and convert many young hearts to the truth."

As she finished her statement I glanced over at Ashley and saw she was beginning to cry. I looked at her with concern.

"What's wrong?"

She looked at both of us.

"Do you smell that?" Ashley asked.

We looked at each other and then back at Ashley.

"No. What?" we both answered at the same time.

We couldn't smell anything.

"It smells like roses in here," Ashley said.

The woman looked at me and I looked at Ashley. We had just finished praying the rosary, and my wife enters the chapel carrying our unborn child and says she can smell roses. It's been said that when one smells roses after praying that means that the Blessed Mother is present. Ashley said she could literally feel her presence.

A week went by and I was becoming very nervous. I had two days remaining at school before I would be taking the week off to welcome my son into the world. I had been informed by John Listi that the scheduled prayer service for Eli was going to be held on the following evening.

The next day at Mass, I was waiting anxiously for

the gospel. I was hoping it would contain the message I had been waiting for, the one that includes the phrase, "Your faith has healed you." I needed to hear those words; I wanted to know that the miracle I had prayed so hard for over the past four months would become a reality.

But that's not the gospel that was read. And I knew, at that moment, Eli would not be born completely normal, but I was okay with that. I know and I accept that God answers our prayers in His way, not ours; in His time, not ours.

After Mass, John invited the student body to the prayer service that was to be held for Eli that night. And toward the end of each of my classes, I invited my students again.

That night in the mall area of the school, the prayer service was held. After John welcomed everyone and played an opening song, I read "Eli's Witness" to the crowd.

It was one of the hardest things I had ever done. I could barely make it through the sentences without breaking down. I could feel the story touching the hearts of all who were in attendance. It was the most meaningful prayer time I had ever had in my life, because I got to share it with my family and many of the students who had lived this with me every day for months.

The following morning, I received an e-mail from a parent who had been in attendance at the prayer service. It read:

Chad,

I wanted to share with you how touched I am by Eli's impending birth, and how thankful I am that Briggs has had you as a teacher this year. You have taught him a lot more than just civics. I hope that he can keep with him forever the lessons you have taught through your actions about being a father and husband.

Sept. 30, 2008, must have been the worst day of your life. But, it seems to me that the process of the past several months has taken you to a place where Feb. 17, 2009, will be one of the happiest days of your life – regardless of the news the day brings.

Hearing you talk last night, I truly came to understand that you have embraced your role as Eli's dad to be one of the many great joys and responsibilities of your life. Eli will be a perfect son, because his parents' love for him is perfect.

Nineteen years ago, my dear friend's son was born with unexpected life-long birth defects. I have always remembered my friend's words as she held her new baby in the hospital after being told the bad news:

"Well, I don't see as how it really makes that much of a difference, really. I love him too much to send him back to where he came from or to wish that he was never conceived. He's perfect to me, really. Just let me know what I need to do to give him the best life possible."

Her words took the air out of the room. And the physician standing there simply responded:

"You've already done it."

I felt privileged to be a part of that moment, and I thought about it last night as you spoke. Your words reminded me so much of the resilient, unwavering love my friend has for her son. He is the second child of three, is now 19, and, even though he is completely deaf and almost blind (among other physical impairments), he speaks and functions at a far higher level than any of the early predictions.

I somehow often think of him as a lucky kid, and think of his parents as fortunate to have him. He is special, and clearly God had a plan for him.

Listening to you last night, I could not help but feel that Eli is a lucky kid, too, and that God has a beautiful plan for him as well. Eli will share a birthday with Michael Jordan, who, after being cut from the basketball team his sophomore year in high school, went on to defy all the odds. I suspect Eli will surprise many as well in ways no one can predict.

God Bless you and your family.

Charlotte Welch

I was touched by Mrs. Welch's letter. It gave me a boost spiritually and psychologically on a pivotal day – my last day of work before I was to welcome Eli into the world.

Chapter 14

Miracle in the classroom

FRIDAY, FEBRUARY 13, WAS MY LAST DAY on campus with my students before heading into the abyss of the unknown. All the anxiety and fear I felt when I first learned of Eli's condition came rushing back. I could feel the nerves in my stomach and the anxiousness of my heart as I pulled into the parking lot that morning.

I had prepared my lesson plans for the substitute teacher who'd be teaching my classes the following week. I had given tests on both my subjects in all five of my classes, and I had a special day planned for my students. I was going to return the tests I had graded, review them with the students, give the students an idea of what they were to do the following week, and make it clear to them the kind of behavior I expected out of them while I was gone.

All of my students knew what was coming, but none knew exactly how to address it. I was going to solve that problem for them that day. I had already decided that I was going to share "Eli's Witness" with all five of my classes. It was to be my way of letting them see a side of me most of them didn't know was there, even though they had gone through this with me for four months or more.

When I read "Eli's Witness" to each class and asked them to pray one last time for Eli before he was born, the response was nothing short of miraculous. I cannot even put into words how much of an impact it seemed to have on my students. I could see it in their eyes that something extraordinary was taking place in their hearts.

As I stood there looking at my seventh-hour class, I was amazed. It was a beautiful Friday afternoon – five minutes after the bell to end the day – and twenty-five sixteen-year-olds were still in the classroom, staring into my soul. I asked them to pray with me one last time for my son. Before I dismissed them I said:

"Thank you for your compassion. I love you, and I will see you when I get back."

Then came a slow rumble of book sacks and footsteps leaving the classroom. A few female students hugged me, and some young men shook my hand and wished me luck.

As I sat in my room at my desk making sure

all the final touches were in order for the following week, I began to write an e-mail to the faculty thanking them for their support and prayers. As I was writing, two of my female students walked up to the front of my desk. It was thirty minutes after class had ended. What they said blew me away. After they left I completed my e-mail to the faculty. Then I wrote a separate one to John Listi. He was going to be the person with whom I kept in contact while we were in New Orleans.

John,

I know I said it to you on Friday, but I wanted to say it again. Thank you for putting together the prayer service for Eli... It is something Ashley and I will never forget. For my family to witness... the support you have given Ashley and me was amazing.

Friday I read aloud to each of my classes "Eli's Witness." John, I wish you could have seen the reaction of the students. It was amazing... Let me give you just a few examples:

• 5th Period, American History – I have a student who has questioned his faith all year long. He would stand to pray but never make the sign of the cross or verbally pray. He has watched me very carefully go through this process, and I know he respects me. Friday, after reading, I asked the class to stand and pray with me one last time for Eli. This guy stood, made the sign of the cross, and prayed! One of his teachers from last year said he didn't know if anything would get to this student. God put him in

my class this year for a reason.

• My seventh-hour class exits stage-right on any day at 2:34 p.m., when the bell rings, like a herd of cows chasing grass. Friday as I attempted to finish reading what I had written, the bell rang. Not one of them moved. They even stayed to pray with me when I finished.

After school, two students came to me at about 3:00 and told me the following:

• Student in 6th hour (junior girl) – "Coach, today when we prayed for your son after you read what you wrote, I could feel God while we prayed. I have felt that way only twice in my life before today. I think you should read that to more people; it would affect them."

• Student in 5th hour (junior girl) – "Coach, I think you should have read that yesterday after Mass. The student body needs to hear that. It would have affected them all."

I just wanted to share this with you... because of our mission. I would never have been ready to face this without what has transpired around that table with you, Father Joe, and all the other guys. It was all preparation for me. I sat at that table one night and told you I just wanted to be a soldier in your army at St. Thomas More to bring kids to Jesus Christ. I believe God has equipped me with something that will allow that mission to obtain unbelievable progress.

Thanks again for being a true friend ....

Know I will feel you praying for us next week.

Love you,
Chad

Chapter 15

Eli's voice

WE GOT AN EARLY START FOR NEW Orleans on Monday February 16. After finishing breakfast with our older son and dropping him off at school, we hit the interstate.

Thoughts of leaving Ephraim with my parents for an indefinite amount of time were running through my mind with every mile marker we passed. I did not know when Ephraim would see his mother again, nor how long Eli would be in the hospital following his birth and the surgery he would need afterward.

I had prepared myself for all of this. But visualizing something and living through it are two different things.

Ashley had an appointment with the doctor who

was going to be delivering Eli. This was only the second time we would be meeting with her. She was in the same field as the specialist we had been seeing in Lafayette, and she had been receiving updates from the Lafayette doctor for several months.

We arrived at the doctor's office at around eleven in the morning. Ashley did not have a firm time for her appointment, but the receptionist said she was going to work us in to see the doctor. It was a good thing for me that I brought some reading material to keep myself occupied, because we did not get to see the doctor until four hours later.

The doctor reassured Ashley and me that everything was going to be okay. We were instructed to arrive at the hospital by six the next morning. I shook the doctor's hand and Ashley and she hugged as we left the office. Ashley said she felt good about the doctor and confident in her ability – which helped me to feel good about the overall situation.

Driving through New Orleans traffic on any given afternoon is challenging all by itself, but to do it while trying to locate a place you have never been is especially stressful. We had good directions, but we were not very familiar with the city. Tulane-Lakeside Hospital is located in Metairie, which is on the outskirts of New Orleans. The couple with whom we were staying, Buddy and Carolyn Kass, lived in Gretna. To get there required our taking I-10 through New Orleans, then crossing the Mississippi River Bridge, then hunting for a particular exit. Thank goodness it was a straight shot and our hosts' home was not far from the exit.

When we arrived, we were pleased to see Ashley's parents' car in the driveway. They were waiting for us. The plan was for them to stay with us through the week. By the weekend, if things with Eli were stable, Ashley's dad and I would return home to Lafayette while Ashley and her mother remained with Eli until he would be released to come home.

The apartment behind the Kass's home was just big enough to hold the four of us and our luggage. After eating supper, showering and watching some television to wind down, we prayed the rosary together before turning the lights out for the night. I slept unusually well that night for being in an unfamiliar bed far from home. It was the last restful night I would have for quite a while.

The following morning, Ashley was admitted to the hospital. A nurse entered her room and prepped her for the impending operation. Ashley requested that in addition to me, her mother be allowed in the operating room during the procedure. In most hospitals only the husbands are allowed to be in the room during a surgical procedure. The room was going to be crowded anyway, because the nurses who were going to take Eli to the neonatal unit were going to be there waiting for him as well. Ashley's mom, Ann, and I were asked to wear scrubs and to wait outside the operating room until a nurse called us in. Ann and I stood in the hallway waiting to be called.

It was a surreal moment. This long, emotional journey was reaching its climax, and it felt like a very long climb from the day of that ultrasound back in September. All the events of the past five months were replaying in my mind when my thoughts were interrupted by the nurse's voice.

"We're ready. You can come in."

The only part of Ashley we could see was her head and her left arm. I sat on a stool next to her and held her hand. The doctor started the Caesarean section procedure. There seemed to be a lot of people doing multiple things all at once. An odd odor filled the room as my wife's incision was being burned by a laser. I could hear the doctor and the head nurse conversing, and as they continued to operate the nurse leaned in and spoke to Ashley.

"You are going to feel some pressure," the nurse said.

Ashley was crying and squeezed my hand so hard I thought it was going to break.

Then I heard it, for the first time: Eli's voice.

He let out a scream. It was one of the most beautiful things Ashley and I had ever heard. All the anxiety of the last five months was gone. Slowly, I began to feel some relief from stress as I heard the nurses in the room saying one after the other:

"The lesion is very small; it's so small."

This was immediately followed by Ann's calm re-assurance as she lifted her hand into view and I saw her index finger and thumb meet to form a small circle.

"It's about the size of a silver dollar," she said.

The opening in Eli's back could have been the size of a saucer, but it wasn't.

The calmness in Ann's voice and in the nurses' voices was like angels whispering in my ear.

Relieved and reassured, I lowered my face into my hands and I began to cry as I silently thanked God. I wiped the tears away as I watched a nurse carry Eli to a table at the foot of Ashley's bed. I got up from my stool and walked around to see him.

"Dad, would you like to cut the cord?" a nurse asked.

"No, thanks," I said.

I was too mentally and physically drained to remain standing, so I returned to my seat. A few minutes later – after they cut the umbilical cord and cleaned him up – one of the nurses walked over to me and slowly placed Eli in my arms.

Although I got to hold him for only about ten seconds, it was an exuberant moment, a heavenly moment. Our son, now out of the womb, now into the world, was squinting in the light, trying to open his eyes. He looked like any healthy baby, with a long, eight-pound frame and perfect soft pinkish skin. He was beautiful. I forgot momentarily that he had ever been diagnosed with anything.

Then as quickly as that heavenly moment came, it was gone as a nurse took him from my arms, placed him in his transport Isolette and rolled him out of the room.

Ashley was taken to a recovery room, and Ann and I went to meet my father-in-law, Randy, in the waiting room. We would have to remain there until Ashley was allowed to have visitors in the recovery room. We would not be able to see Eli until he was stabilized.

I was anxious to drop a line back to my colleagues at St. Thomas More. I had taken my laptop computer with me to try to keep them updated by e-mail. The hospital offered a free wireless internet connection, and I tested it the minute I got to the waiting room. I logged on and saw that I had twenty-six e-mails in my inbox. I tried frantically to answer all of them, but I wore myself out in the process. So I decided to call John and give him a verbal update.

John told me the entire school had stopped to pray around the time Eli was scheduled to be born. Then he asked that I contact him as soon as I knew when Eli's surgery would be. The school community would be praying again just prior to the surgery.

Chapter 16

Eli is going to walk!

THE NEXT THREE DAYS IN THAT HOSPITAL were the longest of my life. On Tuesday evening the neurosurgeon who would be operating on Eli visited my wife and me to inform us that he intended to simultaneously close the lesion in Eli's back and insert a shunt into his head. We were delighted to hear this because originally Eli was supposed to have two separate surgeries. I figured this meant Eli would be home sooner.

The surgeon informed us that the operation was routine and that he didn't anticipate any complications. Ashley seemed satisfied with the meeting with the surgeon and his staff. They talked more to her than to me because they knew she was a nurse and would understand the medical terminology much better than I.

Ashley's parents returned to Gretna for the evening and were planning to come back first thing in the morning for Eli's surgery. I stayed with Ashley in her hospital room. We were allowed to visit Eli in the neonatal unit during certain hours of the day and night. Every couple of hours I was bringing breast milk to my son's nurses so they could continue to feed him. I took Ashley in a wheelchair to see Eli a few times.

Anticipating the surgery was terrible. I could hardly sleep. I was nervous and emotionally exhausted, the portable bed was hard and uncomfortable, and I had to get up every few hours to bring breast milk to the neonatal unit.

Around 6:30 the next morning, Ashley's parents arrived with coffee and breakfast. We were all anxiously waiting to receive word on when the surgery would begin. We sat together and prayed.

We heard a tap on the door, and the neonatal anesthesiologist entered the room. She was there to inform Ashley and me that the surgical team wanted to wait another two days before performing the surgery. An ultrasound showed Eli had two holes in his heart. (I understand this is a very common thing that every infant has while in the womb. The holes usually close up on their own a few days after birth.) The anesthesiologist was afraid that if she administered the anesthesia it might stop the holes from closing up in the normal amount of time. The delay, of course, would prolong our stay in New Orleans.

I began shooting e-mails back to school to let them know what was going on, then I called John to give him the news.

I spent the next two days in prayer, anticipating the procedure which was now scheduled for Friday, February 20. I was aware that it would take about six hours. I figured there would be a series of events that would have to transpire for Eli to be stabilized.

The next two nights sleeping in the hospital beds were not much better than the first. I got up every two hours to bring milk to the neonatal unit. Now able to move around comfortably without the wheelchair, Ashley would walk down the hall to visit with Eli in the unit every few hours.

The next morning around six o'clock we received word that Eli was being wheeled into the operating room. I began praying a novena to the Infant Jesus of Prague, praying that the operation would go well and that Eli would not suffer as a result of it.

We never actually got word from a doctor about Eli's status during or after the procedure, but we were able to see our son after he returned to the neonatal unit. He was sleeping peacefully, and all signs indicated he was going to have a complete recovery.

The next day I was in our apartment in Gretna

and noticed a small statue of the Infant Jesus of Prague. I was stunned when I saw it, and took its presence as a sign that our prayers for Eli's well-being were being answered.

The amount of time Eli remained in the hospital would depend on many factors. The most important thing for Eli to do was to wake up from the operation, begin breathing on his own, eventually start drinking breast milk, and then have a bowel movement.

Ashley was discharged on Saturday afternoon around two o'clock. It was a surreal feeling going to the unit to see Eli, knowing he would not be leaving with us. Now, in order to see Eli each day we were going to have to go back and forth between the hospital in Metairie and the apartment in Gretna.

Eli looked great. He had pulled his breathing tube out of his mouth and was breathing comfortably on his own. He was still being fed through his veins. Our hope was that by the time we returned the following day he would be drinking the milk.

My brother-in-law and his wife had come to visit us and see the baby. They would bring Ashley's dad back to Lafayette that night. Ashley's mom stayed with us. That night I got the first decent night's sleep I had had in five days. The plan for the following morning was to attend 10:30 Mass and then make our way back to the hospital.

Sunday morning, Ashley stayed in bed in the

apartment while her mom and I went to church.

We attended Mass at St. Anthony's, a church connected to a small Catholic school where our hosts did some volunteer work.

As the Mass began, the priest bowed at the altar, took his place facing the congregation, and said something that really got my attention.

"Today, my brothers and sisters, we have a great gospel to reflect on. Jesus heals the paralytic. He says to him, 'Your faith has healed you.'"

I could hardly believe what had just come out of the priest's mouth. This is the very statement I had been hoping to hear the Thursday prior to my son's birth. Now, it was the first Sunday following his birth, and I felt God was speaking to me directly again.

Hearing that gospel, that Sunday, under those circumstances brought my faith to a new level. At that moment, I didn't only hope and believe that Eli will walk someday, I knew it. I clearly, positively knew it. Eli is going to walk!

Now, I could hear for the next twenty years from some of the most brilliant spina bifida specialists in the world that Eli will never walk, and I would not believe them. I don't need a doctor to tell me Eli is going to walk or that he is not going to walk. God has made it clear to me: Eli will walk.

When we returned to the garage apartment after Mass, Ashley was crying. She had found a Mass on television and had heard the same gospel we had.

"Did you hear the gospel today?" I asked excitedly.

"Yes, I did," she replied with a smile.

"Ash, he's going to walk. Eli's going to walk!"

Chapter 17

An emotional roller coaster ride

THE NEXT TWO WEEKS WOULD PROVE to be the most spiritually and emotionally trying since Eli's diagnosis five months earlier. I now faced the reality of being in Lafayette with one son while my wife was in New Orleans with my other son for an undetermined amount of time. I cannot put into words how torn I felt in this situation. It's very stressful – and exhausting – to try to do your job, be a parent, and manage the idea that at any moment you could get a call informing you that you have to be back in New Orleans immediately, although that's physically impossible.

Sunday night I arrived home and was able to pick up around the house and get things in order before Ephraim was brought to me by my parents.

When he arrived, he ran up to me and gave me a huge hug. A little while later my parents accompanied me into his bedroom, and we tucked him in for the night.

"Daddy came home just to see you. I missed you," I told him.

He asked me to lay down with him, and I did. Within five minutes, he was sound asleep. I slept well that night knowing that Eli and Ashley were in good hands and that I was here for Ephraim.

Two days later, on *Mardi Gras* day, I took him to a parade and tried to keep his mind off of his mom. It worked for a good part of the day and into the night. I figured I had only to manage this for another twenty-four hours then Ashley and Eli would be home.

Ashley and I talked at least once a day since I left the past weekend. Eli had been doing so well that he was scheduled to be released from the hospital on February 25, Ash Wednesday, the day after *Mardi Gras*. Originally, he was expected to be in the hospital possibly for a month; now it was looking like he would be home a week and a day following his birth and major surgery. We were overjoyed to learn that our family would be home together in Lafayette very soon.

However, on Wednesday at midday I received a call from Ashley, and she was very upset. She and her mother had packed everything at the apartment in Gretna and had arrived at the hospital only to learn that Eli was going to have to stay longer and would not be released. Another test showed he had developed fluid around his heart. He would have to remain until it cleared up or could be drained. I was very disappointed, too, but I refused to stop believing that all would be well.

"Ashley, it's going to be okay. We just have to keep praying. You both will be home very soon," I said in a confident tone.

I was strong for my wife on the phone, but after hanging up my emotions got the best of me.

I knew my parents would continue to help me with Ephraim, but he had not seen his mom in nearly two weeks. That was beginning to take its toll. Ashley asked me to bring Ephraim to see her that weekend. She missed him. I told her we would leave early Saturday morning and pick up her dad to go with us. He and his wife were going to switch places in the event Ashley and Eli had to stay another week.

The drive on Saturday was pretty smooth, and we arrived at the hospital in Metairie around noon. Ephraim got to visit with his mom and to see his brother for the first time. Children under sixteen are not allowed inside the neonatal unit, so the nurses brought Eli to the window of the door and Ephraim got to take a picture with his little brother. After Ashley fed Eli, we all left and took Ephraim to the Aquarium of the Americas in downtown New Orleans and spent some time together as a family.

Leaving Sunday afternoon was tough on Ephraim – and me, and Ashley. My mother-in-law rode home with Ephraim and me, and she and I had a really good conversation about everything that had transpired. I think we bonded in a way we never had before. Eli's situation was bringing me closer to my wife's family.

It was now the beginning of the first week of March, and I was back at work. I was very busy trying to get caught up on all the work I missed while being out for Eli's birth.

One evening Ashley called to report that the fluid around Eli's heart was gone, but his back had begun leaking spinal fluid. This could be extremely serious. It indicated that possibly his shunt was not working; this could mean a second surgery on his head. The best-case scenario was simply that the stitches in his back – where the doctor had sewed up the lesion – had come loose. This is what the doctors thought had happened.

The following evening, my mother-in-law had come by to drop off Ephraim, and as we were visiting Ashley called. I could tell by the tone of her voice she was very upset.

"They just re-sewed his back, and the doctor said if that does not work he will probably have another surgery. That could put us here another month," Ashley said.

I tried to reassure her that everything would be okay. I was strong for her on the phone, but after hanging up I lost it. My face fell into my hands and I began to cry. I felt as though my faith was being tested again, but I resolved to persevere no matter what the cost.

Wednesday March 4 was the most difficult school day I had that entire year. I opened my first class of the day with an explanation of what was going on with Eli and asked my students to pray a rosary with me before I attempted to teach a lesson. It was beautiful, although I broke down as we were praying. Once again, my students were moved to compassion.

Between classes, I bumped into one of the school administrators in the hallway. He offered a word of encouragement and support.

"I am not going to ask how you're doing. I figure you get asked that too much anyway. I just wanted to let you know, if you need some time we will take care of this. Just let us know," he said.

"Being around my students uplifts me. I don't want any special treatment, but I truly appreciate your concern," I responded as we shook hands.

During the next class period I sent out a school-wide e-mail to ask everyone to pray for Eli, and I explained the scenario my family was facing.

Dear faculty,
Last night at about 8:30 my wife finished talk-ing to the neurologist about Eli. His back had been

sewed up in the first surgery on February 20, and has now begun leaking spinal fluid. The surgeon tried to re-sew his back and re-dressed it last night. If his back does not stop leaking he will more than likely have to have another surgery next week. Ashley was extremely upset because it may keep them in New Orleans for quite some time.

Please take some time today with your students to pray for Eli, but also for our entire family. This is by far the most challenging thing I have ever faced. It has drained me mentally, physically, and emotionally. Christ must be carrying me because my reserves ran out a long time ago. Thanks for your compassion and continued support. It will get better and then we can all share in His (Christ's) Victory.

Peace in Christ,
Chad

As the bell rang for my third-period class, I walked into the classroom and my friend John Listi came in a moment later. He walked up to me and we hugged. I began to cry, and I said, "All I want is for them to come home."

The students entered the room and took their seats. Then I asked them to pray a rosary with me for my son. John stayed, and just as we began praying, our colleague Lance Strother walked in and joined us.

My students witnessed me leaning on two of my brothers in my time of need. They learned much more than just a subject in my classroom this year –

and it was all because of Eli.

In desperation, I sent an e-mail to a friend of mine who I knew could get in touch with Father Manny Fernandez, the healing priest. I was willing to drive to Berwick, pick him up, and take him to the hospital in Metairie so he could pray over Eli. Then I'd turn right back around and bring him back to Berwick. After our experience with Fr. Manny, I knew that if he prayed over Eli no other surgery would be necessary and Eli would come home. Fr. Manny agreed to make the trip, but as it turned out, we didn't need him to go after all.

Wednesday evening I received a phone call from Ashley. Eli had done a complete turn-around, and if everything continued to improve he could be home very soon. I believe Eli's improved condition was the result of the power of prayer.

And on March 6, 2009, Elijah Paul Judice came home for the first time.

Chapter 18

Back to New Orleans

WITH ELI AND ASHLEY HOME NOW, I was finally at peace and able to settle down and concentrate on preparing for a major presentation I was scheduled to give a few days later.

The audience was a Confirmation class at Sacred Heart Church in the nearby town of Broussard. I was the keynote speaker, and my powerpoint presentation dealt with our journey of faith, hope and prayer while waiting for Eli to be born.

Over the past six months, I had shared pieces of this story with many people who seemed to be affected in a positive way by what they were hearing. I believed that, given the opportunity to hear the whole story, from start to finish, many in the audience would gain a new perspective on life, faith, and the power of prayer.

I had spent the past two days putting the finishing touches on the presentation, and I was now prepared to give my testimony. The talk was set for Sunday afternoon, March 8.

The morning of the presentation, I was relaxing on my couch when Ashley walked up to me and placed Eli in my arms. It was the first time I would be able to hold him for any length of time since he was born. As he lay on my chest, he slowly pushed away and raised his head. And our eyes met. It was as though he was looking into my soul, and I into his. I was overwhelmed with joy, and shed a few tears of happiness.

That afternoon, my presentation was well attended by candidates for Confirmation, as well as by my family, friends and colleagues.

The response to the presentation exceeded my expectations. I managed to reach people of all ages. I could see the impact my story had on those in attendance. It had an especially strong impact on two students with whom I had contact on a daily basis.

Several members of the Confirmation class who attended Sacred Heart Church were St. Thomas More students. A good number of them had been in my classroom all year. When I finished my presentation, one of them came up to me and, fighting back tears, he said:

"Coach, I have this huge story to tell you. I didn't

fully get it until today. Can I come by after school tomorrow to talk to you?"

"Sure. I'll see you then," I told him.

A senior from St. Thomas More whom I had become pretty close to through interaction at school was also in attendance. He said:

"Coach, I could not believe it. During your presentation you mentioned a reading from the gospel of Matthew. The woman who had been bleeding for fifty years reached out in faith and grabbed the cloak of Jesus. He turned to her saying, 'Your faith has healed you.' You mentioned that the week before Eli was born that you wanted to hear that reading as the Gospel during the school Mass.

"I just wanted to let you know that the week before Eli was born I went into the chapel to pray every day. I usually prayed for Eli in my daily prayers, but that week I went in there each day with the focus of just praying for him.

"I wasn't sure exactly what to pray for so I tried to find something in the Bible I could reflect on while I prayed for him. I found a picture of him that you left in the chapel and placed it in the Bible next to the reading I chose to reflect on. I read it over and over again and prayed for Eli for fifty minutes each day. Coach, it was *that* reading, the one you wanted to hear.

"I almost started crying when you were talking about it during the presentation. I just wanted to tell you about it. God is amazing."

I was so overwhelmed that I did not know what to say. But I felt that God was using Eli's story to reveal Himself to others.

When I arrived home after the presentation, Ashley was sitting in the den holding Eli, and Ephraim had just come in from playing outside.

"How was it?" she asked.

"Better than I imagined," I said. "That will not be the last time I give that presentation."

We visited with family and friends for the rest of the day and began to try and settle into our new routine. I didn't sleep well that night. I sensed that some kind of storm was coming.

My alarm went off early, then I went to the gym and I struggled through my routine. Emotionally, I was shot, and the recent ordeal had a negative impact on my strength. But that didn't matter much at this point. My thoughts were centered on the fact that my wife and son were now home and now we could begin a new chapter in our lives.

Work that day was going great. Everyone at school had been anticipating Eli's return, and my principal, during the morning announcements, let the entire student body know my boy was home. I was just beginning the lesson with my sixth-period class when my cell phone rang. I noticed it was my wife, then I apologized to my students.

"It's my wife. I have to answer it."

The tone of her voice struck my heart like a dagger.

"Eli's back is leaking. We have to go back to New Orleans. You need to come meet me at home right now," she said as she cried.

I knew my students could hear her frantic tone by the expressions on their faces.

"Everything will be fine. I love you," I said.

I looked at twenty-four teenagers and said:

"I have to go. Pray!"

My principal happened to be in the hall not far from my classroom. I let him know what was transpiring, and he stayed with my class. The people at school were very supportive and assured me everything would be taken care of in my absence. I was in a state of shock as I walked toward my car.

As I drove home I began saying to myself:

"This has to be a dream. We can't possibly have to be going back to New Orleans already. And what about Ephraim?"

That morning Ephraim did not want to go to school because he feared when he returned home we would not be there. Who could blame him? We had been gone for so long, and he had been juggled around so much I don't think he knew where home was anymore. Ashley and I promised him we would be there when he got home. How was he going to react to having his grandparents pick him up again? I didn't have time to dwell on that.

My wife needed me to get her back to New Orleans by five o'clock that afternoon to get Eli started on an antibiotic. Children with spina bifida run a risk of developing spinal meningitis if their wounds become infected.

Now, at this point, my faith was really being tested. We were not even going back to the same hospital. We had to drive into downtown New Orleans, to Tulane Medical Center, where Eli would be admitted to the pediatric unit. Before we left, all I had time to pack was a little luggage and my laptop. I needed a way to stay in contact with my family and with school.

We rushed to the hospital only to have to sit and wait for three hours – like last time. We arrived just prior to five o'clock, but Eli did not get admitted to a room until around eight that night. The medication wasn't given to him until around eleven. After conducting an initial test, one of the doctors suggested that a CT scan was necessary to determine whether the leak was originating in his head or his back.

I stayed in the hospital that night with Ashley and Eli and, naturally, I didn't sleep so well. The next day we waited all day for the results of the CT scan and finally got word sometime after nine o'clock Eli would have to have another operation on his back.

After listening to the doctor's report, I left the

hospital and headed for the apartment in Gretna where we had stayed previously. Ashley stayed in the hospital with Eli. Unfortunately for me, I got lost trying to find my way to the Mississippi River Bridge. I ended up back at the hospital and called the apartment owners, Buddy and Carolyn Kass, apologizing for keeping them up so late waiting for me. They generously offered to come and pick me up, and I accepted without hesitation.

When I got back to the apartment and got ready for bed I realized I had left my cell phone on, and the battery was dead. I had no way of contacting Ashley. I was going to have to wake up early to return to the hospital the following morning because I was catching a ride with one of the Kasses on their way to work.

The only peace of mind I enjoyed was the knowledge that a friend and colleague from Lafayette was coming to meet me the next day to pray at the Shrine of Blessed Father Xavier Seelos. Fr. Seelos was a nineteenth century missionary who moved to New Orleans to treat people who were ill from a yellow fever epidemic. He contracted the disease himself and died after serving the people of the city for about a year. Over the next hundred years or so several miraculous healings were attributed to his intercession.

Wednesday morning I arrived back at the hospital and Ashley was feeding Eli. She gave me an update.

"The doctors came by last night. Eli's shunt is working, and they want to surgically re-sew his back. That's the only explanation for the leaking. He will be rolled into surgery around eleven o'clock," she said, adding, "I tried to call you last night but your phone was dead."

I apologized for the phone problem then told her I would be praying at the shrine during the time of Eli's procedure.

"I can't think of a better place for you to be," she said.

About two hours after this conversation, my colleague, Mary Collins, and her husband, Eddie, arrived from Lafayette. She had attended my presentation to the Confirmation class the previous Sunday and told me how much she enjoyed it. Then she offered her support in my time of trial.

"If there is anything I can ever do for you, just let me know," she said.

Remembering her generous offer, I had called her from New Orleans the day after we arrived and asked her to come to the city and go with me to the Shrine of Fr. Seelos. She readily agreed to make the trip.

Mrs. Collins and I had discussed the powerful intercession of Fr. Seelos, and she had been praying with her class for his intercession on Eli's behalf. Also, she had spoken to me about a life-size statue of Fr. Seelos at the shrine and suggested I should sit down next to him and see what he had to say to me. I was greatly anticipating the moment when I would have such an opportunity.

Chapter 19

An epiphany at the Shrine of Fr. Seelos

W HEN WE ARRIVED AT THE SHRINE OF Blessed Father Seelos in downtown New Orleans, we saw two buildings in a compound, and between them was a paved area, like a courtyard. One building housed a church and the shrine; the other, a gift shop.

We rang the bell at the gift shop and the caretaker of the property greeted us. I told him why we were there.

"My wife is in the hospital with my son, who has spina bifida. We came here today to pray at the shrine for the intercession of Fr. Seelos as my son undergoes his second surgery."

The old man walked us across the courtyard to the shrine. He unlocked the door, and as we entered

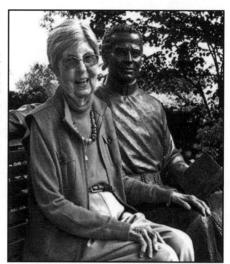

An unidentified visitor to the Shrine of Blessed Father Seelos in New Orleans sits next to the life-size sculpture of the late priest, who is being considered for canonization.

I could see the life-size bronze statue of Fr. Seelos. It was situated on a wooden bench in a seated position. It was turned slightly to the left with his right arm extended over the back side of the bench. It had such a welcoming look – almost as though I was being invited to sit next to him. With his right arm hugging your shoulder, you can lean in and talk to him at close quarters. I sat on the bench with the statue as my companions walked into the church with our guide.

I can't explain the peace I felt as I closed my eyes and began to pray for Fr. Seelos' intercession for Eli. I felt the same way as I did when Ashley and I had met Fr. Manny Fernandez for the first time and were blessed by him. I meditated and tried to hear in the silence of my heart the answer to my questions. Why had God brought Eli back to New Orleans? Why was it necessary for me to be at this place, at this shrine, at this moment? What was the point? As I sat there in silence, I tried to really just listen for an answer.

Then it hit me: I had to come to this place because it was in God's plan all along. The reason I had been allowed to experience all of these things was because God wanted me to share Eli's story with the world. And He knew when this journey began, I just was not ready. I didn't have a strong enough faith; my determination was insufficient. I needed to walk this trying path in order to be ready to take this story to a multitude of people who need to hear it.

The day before we went to the shrine, while I was waiting around during Eli's CT scan, I had sat down with my laptop and started writing the introduction to a book. It would be an attempt to describe all the incredible things that had happened because of Eli's medical condition and his impending birth. I felt a strong impulse to write, so I wrote through the introduction.

However, I wasn't firmly resolved to write a whole book. It seemed like that would be a huge job, a daunting task, and very time-consuming. Given the time it took me to do my full-time job as a school teacher, plus my greatly expanded parenting responsibilities, I didn't have a whole lot of spare time on my hands, to put it mildly.

Still, I felt that telling Eli's story was a sort of responsibility, a duty I could not dismiss without considerable thought. It felt like a calling. And I felt that calling again while I was there, at the shrine, on the bench with the image of Fr. Seelos.

If that was not enough to help me make up my mind to write the book, I heard some strong words of encouragement from my colleague, Mary Collins. After we left the shrine and were in the car headed for lunch, she read the piece I'd written and practically insisted that I keep on writing.

"You've got to tell this story, Chad," she said with excitement in her voice. "You've got to."

After the talk with Mary and the inspiring visit to the shrine, I couldn't wait to get back to the keyboard.

Chapter 20

'A part of something huge'

MARY, EDDIE AND I RETURNED TO THE hospital in the early afternoon after praying at the Shrine of Blessed Father Seelos. We found Ashley in the waiting room. She was tired, somewhat anxious and real hungry.

Ashley was very happy to see the gifts we were bearing: take-out food from one of her favorite New Orleans restaurants, Superior Grill. She wasted no time in beginning her meal.

A few minutes before we arrived, Ashley had been informed that the procedure to re-sew the lesion on Eli's back had been completed successfully and that Eli was being rolled back from the recovery room to his room in the pediatric care area. The surgeon assured us that our son's back would be fine and that he would be able to return home in a day or two.

Meanwhile, my father-in-law was planning to come up the following day with a special car seat that would be used to transport Eli home. I planned to go home the next day, after making sure Eli was okay. Wednesday night, I made my way back to Gretna, without getting lost, and spent my last night in the New Orleans area. The following day, I returned home for Ephraim while Ashley stayed with Eli.

This trip back was much different than the previous one. I felt confident Eli was coming home for good and at the same time I was very concerned about Ephraim. When I got to my parents' to pick up Ephraim, he smiled when he saw me, and I gave him a big hug.

"Daddy, I want to go home," he said.

"We're going home, buddy."

"Are Mommy and Baby Eli home?" he asked.

I couldn't hold back the tears; all the emotion of the past months came rushing back.

"They'll be home really soon," I replied.

As I was backing out of the driveway to go home, Ashley called me and said Eli would be discharged the next day. I could feel in my heart that this part of our journey was ending – and a new one was about to begin.

I returned to school on Friday, March 13. The

day went by rather quickly, and after the bell ending seventh period I had a visitor. This young man was in my fifth-hour American history class. He was also one of the participants at the Confirmation retreat on the previous weekend. He's the guy who approached me after my presentation to the retreatants and said he had "a big story" to tell me one day when I had time. I smiled when he arrived.

"I can't wait to hear this," I said.

"Coach, I wrote it," he said as he handed me a brief diary of sorts.

I began to read it out loud.

> *I am writing this to recognize some of the most amazing people in my life, and how if you truly believe and have patience, miracles do happen.*
>
> *Ever since I was little, I wanted to be a part of something huge, a story I could tell my entire life. I never thought I'd get that opportunity.*
>
> *August 2006 – I am drafted as the new STM Cougar basketball manager. I am terrified to be the only freshman and know absolutely no one.*
>
> *November 2006 – I have become used to the daily routine of basketball. We have a game in Morgan City. We go through the usual tradition: Marshall Kemp buys Skittles, the guys warm up and stretch, and Coach Judice and I take 15 minutes to locate the all-important score book.*
>
> *March 2007 – The basketball season has just ended. I hope to be put in Coach Judice's class next year. This does not happen.*

July 2008 – My father loses his job....

July 2008 (late) – My mother is diagnosed with cancer. She has chemotherapy daily and radiation treatments.

August 2008 – I am put into Coach Judice's American History class....

September 2008 – Hurricane Gustav hits Lafayette and our power goes out for only two hours before coming back on. Dad believes it's an act of God to take care of mom.

September 2008 – My dad is offered a great position at one of Louisiana's most successful companies. My family will be OK.

October 1, 2008 – I miss school this particular Wednesday. I was helping my mom prepare for the arrival of Fr. Emmanuel "Manny" Fernandez and select friends. I had read his book. He is an amazing man, touched by God. My girlfriend, who is also in Coach Judice's class with me, arrived after school and delivered the news of Eli Judice. My mom, Father Manny, and I pray for Eli. One week later, my mom's cancer is completely gone.

December 2008 – Coach Judice tells us Eli has a lot of movement in his lower extremities. This is incredible for a baby with spina bifida. I have a lot of hope for Eli.

February 12, 2009 – I attend a special (prayer service) for Eli and the whole Judice family. I have to say it was the most meaningful praying I've done in my life. All my petty wants and needs were pushed aside to pray for Eli. Coach Judice delivers the best testimony I had ever heard to that point in my life....

February 17, 2009 – Elijah Paul Judice is born....

March 2, 2009 – Eli's back begins to leak fluid. The whole school begins to pray for him. Eli's back soon heals and he needs no surgery.

March 8, 2009 – Coach Judice tops himself with his testimony at my Confirmation retreat that was better than his original. He reveals many facts about his journey with Eli's birth....

March 8, 2008 (later that same evening) – People used to ask me who my heroes were. I never really could give a good answer. Today I realized my hero is Eli. The person who beat all the odds, survived what most don't, and suffered more than most will in our entire lives. His father, Coach Judice, a man who united a whole school in prayer, made a journey many of us will never go on, and took it better than any of us could. And finally my mother, who never complained, never made anyone aware of how much pain she went through.

An underlying theme in my American History class was ordinary people working for a cause bigger than themselves. Those of us in Coach Judice's class no longer needed an example – we are the example....

I don't know why I was lucky enough to witness these overlapping miracles, but I am thankful for the opportunity.... I hope in telling this story about these amazing people in the future it will give people hope, inspiration, and evidence that there is a God and that He cares about us.

I close in saying that the miracles that I witnessed

have jump-started my faith and showed me that God really does still talk to people. You just need to be listening.

– Brennan Joseph Broussard

As I finished reading Brennan's diary, I looked at him and said:

"I just realized you were the only student absent in your class the day I announced something was wrong with Eli. You were with Father Manny and were praying for my son with him before he even knew who we were."

Brennan smiled at me and said:

"Way too many events just line up for this to be a coincidence. It's almost like God set the whole thing up."

"You realize God made sure you were in this class this year," I said.

"Yes, I do," Brennan said with a grin. "Have a great weekend, Coach."

In addition to Brennan's written account, I received an anonymous letter from a student who said Eli's story had affected her in a very positive way – even to the point of restoring her faith in God. I was deeply moved and gratified when I read her letter.

Dear Coach,

I hope to give you comfort in your time of need by telling you my story and your unintentional involvement in it.

My older sister has been my role model since I was a young girl. She hit a rough patch in high school and through her actions and decisions put a strain on my parents' relationship. I had always been a person of little faith, and at this point in time I completely abandoned God and fell into a deep depression.

As the time went on, it only got worse. During my eighth grade year I was cutting class, drinking, smoking, doing drugs, and constantly thinking of killing myself....

My parents divorced last summer, which finally gave me an environment I could adjust to. My depression eventually dispersed, but I never regained my faith in God until this year.

Seeing you face your greatest fear and keeping your faith was inspirational – not asking, "Why me?" but rather asking God for help. This has restored my faith. It is actually stronger than it was before.

I know I can now survive any situation as long as I believe God is with me. I believe this is the purpose of your situation. It is a test of your faith and a way to prove God is always there for us.

I received this letter and the one from Brennan on the same day, Friday March 13 – which made it a very good day. It was made even better by the joyful thought of seeing Ashley and Eli come through the front door, for this was the day they were scheduled to return home to Lafayette, hopefully for good.

Chapter 21

The miracle of Eli's life

WHEN ASHLEY, ELI AND ASHLEY'S DAD arrived at our house around seven o'clock Friday evening, it was one of the happiest moments of my life. Ephraim, too, was beaming, so excited to have his mom home and happy to be able to get close to his little brother.

For the first time, Ashley and I had the sense that Eli was home permanently. We were confident he was going to be fine, now that he was home, now that the operations and the trips to New Orleans were behind us.

But we were still hoping for one more blessing for our newborn son: to have our friend Fr. Manny pray over him and touch him with his healing hands.

About a week after Ashley and Eli's return home, Fr. Manny was scheduled to be at a private residence in Lafayette to pray over a small group of people. Ashley brought Eli and Ephraim to the home and I was able to leave work to join them for a short period of time.

We sat in the den waiting for Fr. Manny to arrive. At one end of the room was a huge picture window that provided a nice view of the back yard. There was also a porch with multiple flower arrangements, a large statue of the Blessed Mother, and several bird feeders hanging right outside the window. It was a beautiful spring day, and the room was lighted by the sunlight that poured in through the window.

When Fr. Manny arrived he took his place at the front of the room, and we made a small semicircle around him. Father went to each person, one by one, and gave his blessing. Then he got to us.

"Father, this is Eli," I whispered.

He smiled to show he recognized us, then he began to pray over Eli. Then he extended his hand to Ephraim, then to Ashley, and finally to me. He touched my forehead and then Eli's. After blessing the last person, he asked us all to hold hands and to join in prayer.

A few days later Ashley and I were taking a walk in our neighborhood. Ephraim was trying to walk our dog and Eli was riding in his stroller. Ashley brought up the subject of getting Eli baptized and reminded me it was my duty to make the arrangements. The conversation drifted to the question of whether only a priest could baptize our son.

"Well, actually, any adult Catholic can baptize someone in the event of an emergency if a priest cannot be found. I have baptized babies at work before because we didn't have a priest available," Ashley said, to my surprise.

I had no idea that she had ever baptized any baby. That was news to me. I was glad to hear it.

The next day, a Saturday, was our fraternity reunion. I rode with my best friend, Kevin Guidry, to meet the rest of our old fraternity brothers.

"I know you've been under a lot of stress lately. I figured this party would be a chance for you to just relax for a while," Kevin said as we headed for the reunion.

"Yeah, I just don't have the energy at this point to explain my situation to anyone else."

"You don't owe anyone an explanation. Just try to have fun," he commented.

So, in the process of trying to have fun, I talked with several of the guys about everything except Eli – work, politics, sports, staying in shape, you name it.

But the small talk shifted to something way more significant toward the end of the reunion when I bumped into a fraternity brother I hadn't seen in years.

He introduced me to his wife, not by my name but as "Ashley's husband," which I found a little odd. Then his wife told me that they had a daughter who had died shortly after birth. I offered my condolences, then she asked me about Eli – which I also found odd since I had never met this woman in my life.

"How do you know about Eli?" I asked.

"My daughter was born at the hospital where your wife works. I have kept in touch with all of the nurses that cared for my daughter. When I last spoke to them and asked specifically about Ashley they informed me of the situation with Eli," she said.

"So, my wife took care of your daughter that died?" I asked.

"Yes, she did, and we will be forever indebted to Ashley," my fraternity brother chimed in.

Then his wife explained to me what had happened six months earlier while Ashley was on duty at the hospital.

"Your wife baptized my child as I held her in my arms before she took her last breath. In fact, when Ashley had completed the sign of the cross on her forehead, she passed. I will never forget your wife, and every time I visit my daughter's grave I pray for your wife."

By now, my heart was in my stomach. I could

hardly believe I was talking to the parents of a child Ashley baptized. It was equally hard to believe that the child's father was my fraternity brother.

Four days after the fraternity reunion, on March 24, my son had a two-week checkup with the neurosurgeon who had preformed his surgeries. The doctor removed the bandages from Eli's back and declared his wound completely healed. He was surprised at the extent of our son's movement of his lower extremities.

That's because the lesion on Eli's back was located at a relatively high point along the spine. Most children with spina bifida whose lesions are that high are not expected to have much movement or feeling from that point on down. But today Eli is moving his legs and his toes and has control of his urine stream and bowels. And one day he is going to walk.

The miracle of Eli's life is not only that he has physical abilities that doctors said he never would, but also that his story has had such a profound impact on the faith and the lives of others – starting with mine.

The dawn is breaking

SINCE ELI CAME HOME FROM THE hospital in mid-March 2009, he's made substantial progress in his early development.

He receives physical therapy four times per month to increase the movement in his legs, and Ashley works with him on practically a daily basis.

In the summer of '09, we received word from a urologist that Eli eventually may be able to be completely potty trained with the aid of medication and without the need for catheterization. He has movement in his lower legs, and he moves his left leg and foot constantly. Although there is less movement in his right leg, he does raise it consistently. The therapists who have worked with him say the motor function of his upper body is age-appropriate and improving daily, and neurologically he is on the same level as any healthy baby of his age.

In September of '09, I was giving Eli a bath and noticed him bending his left knee and pulling his lower leg and foot toward his upper body. Ashley was away from home at the time, so I called her on the phone.

"Have you ever seen Eli bend his knee while you were bathing him?" I asked.

"You must be seeing things," she responded.

Well, then I watched him very closely, but he didn't move his leg again. So, I thought maybe Ashley was right. Maybe it was just my imagination.

However, a few days later, Ashley and I were both home and I was giving Eli his bath, and I saw him do it again. He bent his knee and brought his leg out of the water toward his upper body. I called Ashley in from the next room.

"Ashley, come see!" I said excitedly.

The second she walked through the bathroom door, he did it again. Her eyes met mine after she witnessed the movement, and her hand covered her mouth as she began to cry.

"Did you see it?" I asked.

Choked with emotion and unable to speak, she nodded as tears of joy streamed down her face.

As we approached Christmas of 2009, Eli was nearly able to sit upright on his own, but he still needed a little support to keep his back straight and his chest out. Faith tells me this will come in time.

I also saw him stand upright for the first time in his life. This is because of a unique piece of equipment designed for children with spina bifida. It is called a "stander" and it looks like a modified wheelchair. Ephraim calls it "Eli's chariot." Eli's hands reach the tops of the wheels of his stander, and he is learning how to move the wheels in two directions, forward and backward. I watched him try to move the wheels in my direction as I kneeled in front of him with tears welling up in my eyes. I beckoned him to come forward, as every father does while coaxing his son to take his first steps.

I am frequently asked about our son's condition. I normally respond by saying he is doing better than the doctors ever expected. Then I add with emphasis that what is so beautiful about Eli is his smile. When my eyes meet his I feel like he is staring into my soul. I can truly feel God's presence in his life. Ashley and I have come to realize the gift we have been given in this little guy named Eli.

In the time since Eli's birth I have shared his story with as many people as possible, as I promised God I would. I have spoken to groups of people of all ages, to crowds ranging from thirty to a thousand.

I am gratified by the audiences' response, which has been overwhelmingly positive and welcoming. (See Appendix 2) I plan to keep on telling Eli's story, not only in my home state of Louisiana but all over the United States and in any venue where I will be welcomed. I believe this story demonstrates the power of prayer and the profound value of all human life.

I also believe Eli's story has only just begun.

Eli's Witness

(A Father's Reflection)

Four years ago (2005) as I was leaving Cathedral-Carmel School and preparing to begin my career at St. Thomas More, I had just witnessed the birth of my first son, Ephraim. Overwhelmed by the challenges of parenting, yet overjoyed at the fact that my ultimate goal in my career was finally being fulfilled (i.e., teaching at St. Thomas More), I was asked a peculiar question by a student in my eighth grade class.

"What is your greatest fear?"

My life was perfect, or so it seemed, and I had never really thought about my greatest fear. But then an answer came to me as clear as day. (I should tell you I am the quintessential perfectionist; everything I do is done very methodically and always has a disciplined structure. I have been that way my whole life.)

So, I told the student that my greatest fear in life would be to have a child born with a physical or mental handicap – because I didn't think, being a perfectionist, I could handle that very well.

After that day, I never gave my response a second thought. The following year I began teaching at St. Thomas More.

Then, on September 30, 2008, my greatest fear became my reality.

A scheduled twenty-week ultrasound revealed that my second son was diagnosed with spina bifida. That day, that moment, was the worst of my life. It is a rare spinal disorder that affects many aspects of a person's everyday life.

My wife, Ashley, who is a nurse and cares for premature babies, knew the severity of the situation upon diagnosis. Feeling an emptiness inside like I had never felt before, I called someone who we had become very close to in my three years at St. Thomas More: Father Joe Breaux, pastor of Saint Alphonse in nearby Maurice. He arrived at our home to offer comfort and consolation to Ashley and me. He asked me what my immediate feelings and reactions were. I responded by saying I was scared. Fear of the unknown will test one's faith beyond description.

How would this affect my marriage? How would it affect my relationship with my first son? How would it affect my son's relationship with his brother? Would it affect our financial capability to pay for their planned Catholic education? How were we going to manage the astronomical medical bills that would accompany this dreaded birth defect? These questions, I have learned in the past months, can be answered only through faith.

Ashley and I sat alone in our house as she read the information the specialist gave us on our unborn son's condition. With tears rolling down her face, she looked at me in a moment of weakness.

"I am going to hell. I am actually thinking about aborting this child," she said.

What would make any mother think this?

Statistical studies show that eighty percent of the people who have knowledge prior to birth that their child has spina bifida choose abortion. Seventy-five percent of the pregnancies result in miscarriages before twenty weeks of pregnancy. The possibility that your child will never walk, nor have control of his bowel movements, is a pretty depressing thought.

Fear could have guided our decision, but it didn't. Faith did! I held my wife by the shoulders and said:

"We need to trust God the way Ephraim trusts in us."

My words to her were a direct reference to the Gospel of Matthew 18:2-5:

> *He called a little child and had him stand among them. And he said, "I tell you the truth, unless you change and become like children you will never enter the kingdom of heaven. Therefore, whoever humbles himself like this child is the greatest in the kingdom of heaven. And whoever welcomes a little child like this in my name welcomes me."*

We chose life for our son, who we believe has a purpose that in many ways is already beginning to be revealed to us and to the world. Our childlike trust in God the Father has given us peace and consolation in our deepest suffering and despair.

The next day at a regular school Mass, the priest rose to proclaim the gospel. As the words he read aloud were the same I had referenced the night before to my wife, I felt God was acknowledging the fact that we turned to Him and not to the darkness. He seemed to be saying,

"Fear not the world, for I have conquered it, and with that conquered your fear. Have faith in me, and I will deliver you."

Everyone present remembers what my friend, John Listi, did after Mass. He announced to the school community my son's condition and asked twelve hundred students, faculty, staff and parents to pray for a miracle.

I have witnessed firsthand many miracles from that time to the present, and this summer I will undertake the challenge of sharing them with the world. My prayer for Eli and our family began that day and will continue for the rest of my life. My life has, in many ways, become a constant prayer. This is where my strength lies.

Since October 2008, I have prayed daily in the chapel at St. Thomas More High School. I have prayed with parents of students who attended our school. I feel that God speaks to me through them daily.

Faith has saved my family, and I know it will save Ephraim and Eli. Whether Eli is born completely healthy or not, it doesn't matter, for he is a miracle. So my prayer has already been answered.

Peace in Christ,
Coach Judice

APPENDIX 2

Public reaction to Eli's story

Following are a few of the letters I received from people who heard and saw my presentation of Eli's story. The responses came after my talks at Catholic high schools in Lafayette, La., mostly in September of 2009.

Chad,

The response from the teachers this morning has been overwhelming. They loved our Day of Reflection. Teachers who have been here over 25 years told me it's the best one we have ever had!

You bared your soul and truly touched them. Continue to answer God's call to share your story.

– *Jill Spikes*
Cathedral-Carmel School

* * *

I can't tell you how much I enjoyed your testimony yesterday. People have been talking about it ever since... very, very powerful, just as I thought it would be. But until you actually hear the story and the amazing little miracles associated with your journey, one can't really appreciate it!

God bless...

Jane Deblieux
Cathedral-Carmel School

* * *

I wanted to send you an e-mail saying how AWE-SOME your testimony was last night! Very moving and powerful!... It has changed my viewpoint on a lot of things and has made me realize that I need to be closer to God.

I have been slacking lately in going to church, but after last night I told myself this is God talking to me and I need to listen!

My mom passed away when I was 15 years old and there is not one day that I don't think about her. When I heard the day Eli was born I broke down even harder – because Feb. 17 is my mom's birthday, too.

So, I just wanted to say a big "thank you" to you and Eli! Your journey has made me realize what I have been missing out on: a relationship with God!

– *Jill Stoute*
(Family friend)

* * *

I heard about your son last year with the rest of the school. I don't know why, but I felt like I needed to help.

I never really went to church and prayed or anything, but I do believe in God and miracles. I started going to church for Eli. I prayed for him as often as I thought of him.

I only knew as much about Eli as my teachers briefly told us. I wanted to learn more so I went to your testimony tonight. It was one of the most moving stories I had ever heard.

One moment that I know I will never forget is when you were talking about Father Manny. My boyfriend was sitting on the left of me and my best friend on my right. As soon as you started talking about Father Manny, my body felt like it was on fire, literally. I was burning up and I thought I was going to faint. As soon as you changed the subject I was cool again. After your testimony I asked my boyfriend and my friend if they felt it. My boyfriend is over 200 lbs., so if it was just hot in the room, he most certainly would've felt it, but he didn't. My best friend, on the other hand, felt the exact thing as me. We always have gotten messages from God while we were together. (It's kind of weird but really cool!)

Once I got home, I went straight to my mom and told her what happened. She told me that my grandmother used to go see Father Manny often, so I called her. She told me that she and my grandfather would go on special trips to go see Father Manny, and on one of the trips my grandfather's rosary had turned gold, just like yours....

Your son, Eli, is an amazing baby. He changed my life while still in the womb! I can only imagine how many lives he will change now that he is in the world.... He is loved by so many and you're a blessed father to have such a powerful son.

I hope I didn't waste your time by sending this, but I felt it was important to tell you how you and your son saved my soul. Eli's story showed me how to value life and my faith.

Thank you.

Jessica Willis
Class of 2010
St. Thomas More High School

*   *   *

You rocked our world!

Students were talking about your testimonial as they were picking up their bookbags from the classroom.

It was after dismissal and on their own time, but they were still talking about it. Some cried, others remained quiet. All were touched.

Thank you. I have kept all of your e-mails (I was in Claire's regiment of the Eli Prayer Army, so she shared them as she received them.) Although I know you and knew most of your story, I felt the true passion of it this afternoon as you spoke of yours and Ashley's journey. Very powerful! All of us appreciate your sharing your story with us at Teurlings Catholic High School.

Smiles & Cheer,

Aline Norwood
Development Director
Teurlings Catholic High School

*   *   *

Words cannot express our gratitude for taking time out of your very busy schedule to share your story with our school! I was deeply moved along with everyone in the gym yesterday. You speak with such passion and conviction that you make it difficult NOT to want to deepen your faith and trust with ALL your heart. Thank you.

Coach Sonny Charpentier told me this morning that after football practice yesterday a group of seniors approached him wanting to hold a prayer service today after school for their teammate whose mother has Stage 4 cancer. Coach Sonny commented that that rarely happens and that he believes they were deeply moved by your testimony and the power of prayer! The prayer service is this afternoon and Eli will be included.

I spoke with several other students after you left who said you were "awesome." I could tell they were filled! We dedicated our Mass this morning to Eli and your entire family and will continue to pray for you along your journey....

Please know we are continuing to pray for continued good health of Eli and for strength for you, Ashley and Ephraim.

Thank you again, and God bless.

Ramey Badeaux
Campus Minister
Teurlings Catholic High School

Index

Indexer's note: Page references in *italics*
refer to photographs and illustrations.

About the Author...

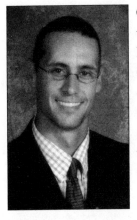

CHAD JUDICE is a high school teacher of civics and American history at St. Thomas More Catholic High School in Lafayette, Louisiana. He began teaching there in 2005 after teaching and coaching basketball the previous four years at Cathedral-Carmel, another Catholic school in Lafayette.

He was nominated several times for the Lafayette Education Foundation Teacher of the Year Award, including once in the Inspirational Category.

He earned a Bachelor of Science degree in Secondary Education Social Studies from the University of Louisiana at Lafayette in 2001. He is married to Ashley (nee) Guillotte, and they have two small children, Ephraim and Eli. They make their home in Lafayette.

Inspiring Books
from
Acadian House Publishing

Waiting For Eli
A Father's Journey

A 176-page hardcover book about a Lafayette, La., couple and their infant son Eli who was born with a dreaded birth defect called spina bifida. It is an inspiring story of faith, hope and the power of prayer. The book takes us on an emotional roller coaster ride, starting with the day the author first learns of his son's medical condition. This moving story has a strong pro-life, pro-love message, and is made even more compelling by the author's descriptions of little miracles along the way. (Author: Chad Judice. ISBN: 0-925417-65-3. Price: $16.95)

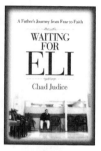

Dying In God's Hands

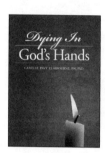

A 152-page hardcover book that provides keen insights into the hearts and minds of the dying. It is based on a dozen or more interviews with terminally ill hospice patients, in which they share their hopes, dreams, fears and needs. The majority of the interviews provide evidence that faith in God and belief in the hereafter are the greatest strengths of the dying. Designed to comfort the dying and their loved ones, the book also contains a section of prayers and prose from all major world religions. (Author: Camille Pavy Claibourne. ISBN: 0-925417-64-5. Price: $16.95)

Water From Stones
An Inner Journey

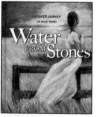

A 128-page hardcover book that is designed to serve as an instrument of healing, renewal and enlightenment for those who are seeking to walk a spiritual path. It is a book for those who are willing to take positive steps toward a more meaningful, more joyful life. The author maintains that the events and circumstances that test our hearts and spirits can bring forth our greatest gifts. She points out that spiritual and psychological healing comes to us as we learn and accept what she refers to as "the lessons of the desert." (Author: Lyn Holley Doucet. ISBN: 0-925417-40-8. Price: $12.95)

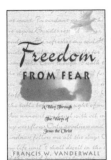

Freedom From Fear
A Way Through The Ways of Jesus The Christ

Everyone at one time or another feels fear, guilt, worry and shame. But when these emotions get out of control they can enslave a person, literally taking over his or her life. In this 142-page softcover book, the author suggests that the way out of this bondage is prayer, meditation and faith in God and His promise of salvation. The author points to the parables in the Gospels as Jesus' antidote to fears of various kinds, citing the parables of the prodigal son, the good Samaritan, and the widow and the judge. Exercises at the end of each chapter help make the book's lessons all the more real and useful. (Author: Francis Vanderwall. ISBN: 0-925417-34-3. Price: $14.95)

Grand Coteau
The Holy Land of South Louisiana

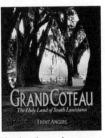

A 176-page hardcover book that captures the spirit of one of the truly holy places in North America. It is a town of mystery, with well-established ties to the supernatural, including the famous Miracle of Grand Coteau. Brought to life by dozens of exceptional color photographs, the book focuses on the town's major religious institutions: The Academy of the Sacred Heart, Our Lady of the Oaks Retreat House and St. Charles College/Jesuit Spirituality Center. The book explores not only the history of these three institutions but also the substance of their teachings. (Author: Trent Angers. ISBN: 0-925417-47-5. Price: $44.95)

Blessed Be Jazz
The Story of My Life as a Clarinet-Playing Jesuit Priest in The French Quarter of New Orleans

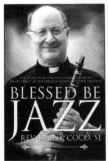

The 192-page hardcover autobiography of Rev. Frank Coco, SJ (1920-2006), a Jesuit priest who served for more than 50 years in south Louisiana as a retreat director, high school teacher and jazz musician. Using his clarinet, he performed extensively in New Orleans nightclubs, sitting in with some of the best-known jazz musicians of his time, including Ronnie Kole, Al Hirt and Pete Fountain. (Author: Rev. Frank Coco, SJ. ISBN: 0-925417-89-0. Price: $19.95)

An Airboat on the Streets of New Orleans
A Cajun couple lends a hand after Hurricane Katrina floods the city

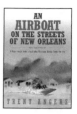

A 192-page book about a Cajun couple from Breaux Bridge, La., who took their airboat into New Orleans when the city flooded as a result of Hurricane Katrina. Doug Bienvenu, the airboat operator, and Drue LeBlanc, who was suffering with kidney disease, rescued hundreds of people during their 3-day mission of mercy. (Author: Trent Angers. Hardcover ISBN: 0-925417-87-4. Price: $16.95. Softcover ISBN: 0-925417-88-2. Price: $14.95.)

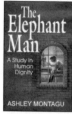

The Elephant Man
A Study in Human Dignity

The Elephant Man is a 138-page softcover book whose first edition inspired the movie and the Tony Award-winning play by the same name. This fascinating story, which has touched the hearts of readers throughout the world for over a century, is now complete with the publication of this, the Third Edition. Illustrated with photos and drawings of The Elephant Man. (Author: Ashley Montagu. ISBN: 0-925417-41-6. Price: $12.95.)

Dreaming Impossible Dreams
Reflections of an Entrepreneur

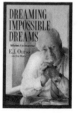

This 176-page autobiography is the rags-to-riches story of multimillionaire philanthropist E.J. Ourso of Donaldsonville, Louisiana, the man for whom the LSU Business School is named. It reveals how Ourso acquired 56 businesses in 48 years – the first 25 with no money down. A testament to the effectiveness of the American free enterprise system, the book chronicles Ourso's life beginning with his early years as a salesman. It reveals his secrets to the acquisition of wealth. (Author: E.J. Ourso with Dan Marin. Hardcover ISBN: 0-925417-42-4, Price $22.95; Softcover ISBN: 0-925417-43-2, Price $16.95)

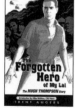

The Forgotten Hero of My Lai
The Hugh Thompson Story

A 248-page hardcover book that tells the story of the U.S. Army helicopter pilot who risked his life to rescue South Vietnamese civilians and to put a stop to the My Lai massacre during the Vietnam War in 1968. An inspiring story about the courage to do the right thing under extremely difficult circumstances, regardless of the consequences. Illustrated with maps and photos. (Author: Trent Angers. ISBN: 0-925417-33-5. Price: $22.95)

TO ORDER, list the books you wish to purchase along with the corresponding cost of each. Add $3 per book for shipping & handling. Louisiana residents add 8% tax to the cost of the books. Mail your order and check or credit card authorization (VISA/MC/AmEx) to: Acadian House Publishing, Dept. B-57, P.O. Box 52247, Lafayette, LA 70505. Or call (800) 850-8851. To order online, go to www.acadianhouse.com.